AF577077

The Institute of Mathematics and its Applications Conference Series

Previous volumes in this series were published by Academic Press to whom all enquiries should be addressed. Forthcoming volumes will be published by Oxford University Press throughout the world.

NEW SERIES

1. *Supercomputers and parallel computation* Edited by D. J. Paddon
2. *The mathematical basis of finite element methods*
   Edited by David F. Griffiths
3. *Multigrid methods for integral and differential equations*
   Edited by D. J. Paddon and H. Holstein
4. *Turbulence and diffusion in stable environments* Edited by J. C. R. Hunt
5. *Wave propagation and scattering* Edited by B. J. Uscinski
6. *The mathematics of surfaces* Edited by J. A. Gregory
7. *Numerical methods for fluid dynamics II*
   Edited by K. W. Morton and M. J. Baines
8. *Analysing conflict and its resolution* Edited by P. G. Bennett
9. *The state of the art in numerical analysis*
   Edited by A. Iserles and M. J. D. Powell
10. *Algorithms for approximation* Edited by J. C. Mason and M. G. Cox
11. *The mathematics of surfaces II* Edited by R. R. Martin
12. *Mathematics in signal processing*
    Edited by T. S. Durrani, J. B. Abbiss, J. E. Hudson, R. N. Madan, J. G. McWhirter, and T. A. Moore
13. *Simulation and optimization of large systems*
    Edited by Andrzej J. Osiadacz
14. *Computers in mathematical research*
    Edited by N. M. Stephens and M. P. Thorne
15. *Stably stratified flow and dense gas dispersion*
    Edited by J. S. Puttock
16. *Mathematical modelling in non-destructive testing*
    Edited by Michael Blakemore and George A. Georgiou
17. *Numerical methods for fluid dynamics III*
    Edited by K. W. Morton and M. J. Baines
18. *Mathematics in oil production*
    Edited by Sir Sam Edwards and P. R. King
19. *Mathematics in major accident risk assessment*
    Edited by R. A. Cox
20. *Cryptography and coding*
    Edited by Henry J. Beker and F. C. Piper
21. *Mathematics in remote sensing*
    Edited by S. R. Brooks
22. *Applications of matrix theory*
    Edited by M. J. C. Gover and S. Barnett

Continued overleaf

23. *The mathematics of surfaces III*
Edited by D. C. Handscomb
24. *The interface of mathematics and particle physics*
Edited by D. G. Quillen, G. B. Segal, and Tsou S. T.
25. *Computational methods in aeronautical fluid dynamics*
Edited by P. Stow
26. *Mathematics in signal processing II*
Edited by J. G. McWhirter
27. *Mathematical structures for software engineering*
Edited by Bernard de Neumann, Dan Simpson, and Gil Slater
28. *Computer modelling in the environmental sciences*
Edited by D. G. Farmer and M. J. Rycroft
29. *Statistics in medicine*
Edited by F. Dunstan and J. Pickles

Statistics in Medicine

Based on the proceedings of a conference on Applications of Statistics in Medicine organized by The Institute of Mathematics and its Applications and held at the University of Wales College of Cardiff in April 1988

Edited by

F. DUNSTAN
University of Wales College of Cardiff

J. PICKLES
National Power plc, Surrey

CLARENDON PRESS · OXFORD · 1991

Oxford University Press, Walton Street, Oxford OX2 6DP
Oxford New York Toronto
Delhi Bombay Calcutta Madras Karachi
Petaling Jaya Singapore Hong Kong Tokyo
Nairobi Dar es Salaam Cape Town
Melbourne Auckland
and associated companies in
Berlin Ibadan

Oxford is a trade mark of Oxford University Press

Published in the United States
by Oxford University Press, New York

British Library Cataloguing in Publication Data
(Data available)

Library of Congress Cataloging in Publication Data
(Data available)

ISBN 0–19–853662–3

Printed in Great Britain by Bookcraft (Bath) Ltd
Midsomer Norton, Avon

PREFACE

This IMA Conference on the applications of statistics to medicine sought to bring together some of the newer topics which have developed since the earlier 1975 conference. We considered new work in the areas of hypothesis testing, epidemiological modelling and prediction, computational tools and diagnostic applications.

The hypothesis testing talks focussed on the still unresolved question of the contribution of low doses of ionising radiation to excess cancer rates in individuals or clusters of leukaemia cases in the community. Darby and Wakeford et al showed some of the detailed investigation needed, and some of the pitfalls of over-hasty analysis, or "trial by TV". The contrasting paper by Openshaw gave an account of a new 'Geographical Analysis Machine' as a technique for hypothesis trawling.

There were several contributions in the area of epidemiological modelling. Griffiths and Reece described models for the spread of AIDS. They showed their potential as predictive tools to help, for example, health service resourcing as well as showing some facets of the numerical mathematics needed. Palmer gave a more qualitative but very colourful description of practical experience in breaking down sources of food poisoning outbreaks, both in the U.K. and abroad while Duffy et al showed how to link descriptive and analytical techniques in an interesting application to cancer epidemiology in the rapidly changing life patterns in Singapore.

The first day's programme concluded with two more theoretically oriented papers. Pickles and Crouchley described the use of stochastic models, compared with more conventional data analysis, as a means of gaining understanding of the parent/child interaction in psychiatric and foster-placement applications. Hughes and Pocock developed a Bayesian approach for the refinement of 'stopping rules' in clinical trials, to achieve the ethically important objective of allowing patients to benefit from information gained during the course of a trial.

The impact of the 'expert systems' approach was shown in the paper by Ashford, who described the practical implementation of a patient/prescription data base system and its natural extensions to more 'intelligent' modes of operation.

The final session of the conference was devoted to a set of papers showing the practical impact of statistical techniques to problems of medical diagnosis and prognosis. Patterson et al showed how discriminant analysis and signal processing could be combined in a practical system for diagnosing hip dislocation in small babies. Discriminant analysis was also used by Jerwood et al for the prognosis of severe head injuries. Here, as in the application of correspondence analysis to diagnosis of chest pain, described by Crichton and Hinde, prompt decision making is vital for the care of the patient. The final two papers covered applications to the detection of blood clots in orthopaedic patients (Kernohan et al) and a multivariate model interpretation of glucose tests in diabetics (Farrow), emphasising the very wide range of statistical techniques available and medical needs in this expanding subject area.

J. Pickles,
National Power Plc

F. Dunstan
University of Wales
College of Cardiff

ACKNOWLEDGEMENTS

The Institute thanks the authors of the papers, the editors, Dr. J. Pickles (National Power PLC, Surrey) and Dr. F. Dunstan (University of Wales College of Cardiff)and also Miss Pamela Irving, Miss Deborah Brown, Miss Donna Smith, Mrs Anne Harding and Miss Karren Robinson for typing the papers.

CONTENTS

CONTRIBUTORS

J.R. ASHFORD; *Exeter Health Information Services Ltd., Thornlea, New North Road, Exeter, EX4 4JZ.*

F.B. BRADLEY; *Queen's University of Belfast, Department of Orthopaedic Surgery, Musgrave Park Hospital, Belfast, BT9 7JB, Northern Ireland.*

J.G. BROWN; *Queen's University of Belfast, Department of Orthopaedic Surgery, Musgrave Park Hospital, Belfast, BT9 7JB, Northern Ireland.*

K. BINKS; *British Nuclear Fuels plc, Warrington, Cheshire.*

N.J. CRICHTON; *Department of Mathematical Statistics and Operational Research, University of Exeter, Rennes Drive, Exeter, EX4 4PU.*

R. CROUCHLEY; *Department of Sociology, University of Surrey, Guildford, GU2 5XH.*

S.D. DARBY; *Imperial Cancer Research Fund Cancer Epidemiology Unit, University of Oxford, Gibson Laboratories, Oxford, OX2 6HE.*

S.W. DUFFY; *MRC Biostatistics Unit, 5 Shaftesbury Road, Cambridge, CB2 2BW.*

M. FARROW; *Department of Mathematics & Computer Studies, Sunderland Polytechnic, Priestman Building, Green Terrace, Sunderland, SR1 3SD.*

F.A. GEORGIAKODIS; *Graduate School of Industrial Studies, University of Piraeus, 40 Karaoli-Dimitriou Street, Piraeus, Greece.*

L. GOURLEY; *Department of Community, Occupational and Family Medicine, National University of Singapore, Singapore.*

J.D. GRIFFITHS; *University of Wales College of Cardiff, School of Mathematics, Senghenydd Road, Cardiff, CF2 4AG.*

J.P. HINDE; *Department of Mathematical Statistics and Operational Research, University of Exeter, Rennes Drive, Exeter, EX4 4PU.*

M.D. HUGHES; *Department of Epidemiology and Population Sciences, London School of Hygiene and Tropical Medicine, Keppel Street (Gower Street), London, WC1E 7HT.*

D. JERWOOD; *School of Mathematical Sciences, University of Bradford, Richmond Road, Bradford, West Yorkshire, BD7 1DP.*

W.D. KERNOHAN; *The Queen's University of Belfast, Department of Orthopaedic Surgery, Musgrave Park Hospital, Belfast, BT9 7JB, Northern Ireland.*

H.P. LEE; *Department of Community, Occupational and Family Medicine, National University of Singapore, Singapore.*

A.H. LEYLAND; *Department of Mathematics & Computer Studies, Sunderland Polytechnic, Priestman Building, Green Terrace, Sunderland, SR1 3SD.*

R.A.B. MOLLAN; *The Queen's University of Belfast, Department of Orthopaedic Surgery, Musgrave Park Hospital, Belfast, BT9 7JB, Northern Ireland.*

S. OPENSHAW; *Centre for Urban and Regional Development Studies, The University of Newcastle-upon-Tyne, Newcastle-upon-Tyne, NE1 7RU.*

S.R. PALMER; *Welsh Unit of CDSC, Cardiff Royal Infirmary, Newport Road, Cardiff, CF2 1SZ.*

C.C. PATTERSON; *Department of Community Medicine & Medical Statistics, The Queen's University of Belfast, Institute of Clinical Science, Grosvenor Road, Belfast, BT12 6BJ.*

A. PICKLES; *MRC Child Psychiatry Unit, Institute of Psychiatry, DeCrespigny Park, London, SE5 8AF.*

S.J. POCOCK; *Department of Epidemiology and Population Sciences, London School of Hygiene and Tropical Medicine, Keppel Street (Gower Street), London, WC1E 7HT.*

D.J. PRICE; *Department of Neurosurgery, Pinderfields Hospital, Wakefield, West Yorkshire, WF1 4DG.*

G. REECE; *Department of Engineering Mathematics, Queen's Building, University Walk, Bristol, BS8 1TR.*

R. WAKEFORD; *British Nuclear Fuels plc, Warrington, Cheshire.*

P.E. WARD; *The Queen's University of Belfast, Department of Orthopaedic Surgery, Musgrave Park Hospital, Belfast, BT9 7JB, Northern Ireland.*

K.A. WHEELER; *University of Wales College of Cardiff, School of Mathematics, Senghenydd Road, Cardiff, CF2 4AG.*

D. WILKIE; *UK Atomic Energy Authority, Seascale, Cumbria.*

A RECENT STUDY OF THE HEALTH OF UK ATMOSPHERIC NUCLEAR WEAPON TEST PARTICIPANTS

Sarah C. Darby
(Imperial Cancer Research Fund Cancer Epidemiology Unit, Gibson Laboratories, University of Oxford)

A follow-up study has recently been carried out of the health of men who participated in the UK atmospheric nuclear weapon tests and experimental programmes that were carried out in Australia and the Pacific between 1952 and 1967. The study was carried out jointly between NRPB and ICRF, and full details have been reported elsewhere.[1,2]

In order to carry out the study, the names of men who participated in the tests were identified from archives of the Ministry of Defence and a matched control group was selected from the same archives. The study groups thus defined totalled 22,347 partipants and 22,326 controls. Men in both groups were followed up using the National Health Service Central Registers at Southport and Edinburgh. Ninety-nine point six per cent were traced to 1 January 1984 and the rates of mortality and cancer incidence (as determined from death certificates and national records of cancer registration) were compared in the two groups. The numbers of deaths observed were also compared with those that would have occurred if the men had experienced the death rates recorded for all men of the same ages over the same years in England and Wales.

No comprehensive list of test participants had been compiled at the time of the tests and it could not be assumed that all participants had been identified during the course of the study. Names of participants and identifying details were, therefore, also sought from many other sources. Reports were received of 2161 individuals who were apparently eligible for inclusion and who were adequately identified, and these 'independent respondents' were followed as a separate group. Of these, 1707 had already been included in the main study group, 414 were accepted as participants but had not been included, and 7 could not be traced in MOD records.

Altogether 3198 deaths were recorded in the two main study groups and the certified cause of death was determined for 3134 (98.0%). Mortality rates in the two groups were closely similar, the relative risk (RR) in the participants compared with the controls being 0.96 for neoplasms, 1.00 for other known non-violent causes, 1.07 for accidents and violence, and 1.01 for all causes. In both groups the mortality was less than expected from national rates, the standardised mortality ratios (SMRs) being respectively 80 and 83 for neoplasms and 80 and 79 for all causes. In the main analyses, thirty eight causes of death were examined. In 6 cases the mortality rates in participants and controls differed significantly at the 5% level (by one-sided tests). Mortality from leukaemia (p=.004), multiple myeloma (p=.009) and 'other injury and poisoning' (p=.04) was higher in the participants and mortality from cancer of the prostrate (p=.01), cancer of the kidney (p=.02) and chronic bronchitis, emphysema, and chronic obstructive lung disease (p=.02) was higher in the controls. Examination of cancer incidence rates showed similar differences for leukaemia (p=.009), multiple myeloma (p=.0007) and cancer of the kidney (p=.01), but different results for cancer of the prostrate, for which the rates were about equal in both groups, and for cancer of the lung, for which the rate was higher in the controls (p=.03). Examination of the rates from cancer in different groups of participants, divided according to measured doses of external irradiation and different types of participation, failed to show any relationship between leukaemia, multiple myeloma, or all neoplasms and the recorded doses of external radiation, and it showed very little difference between the experience of different groups of participants. The highest RRs and SMRs for leukaemia and multiple myeloma were observed in men who were <u>not</u> present at a major test or involved in minor trials at Maralinga. A study of the 11 participants in this group who developed multiple myeloma or leukaemia (other than chronic lymphatic leukaemia) and 33 other participants in the same group matched for age failed to indicate any specific risk factor.

The difference between the two groups in the mortality from leukaemia and multiple myeloma was largely due to extraordinarily low rates from these diseases in the controls (SMRs respectively of 32 and 0), while the mortality in the participants was only slightly greater than expected from national rates (SMRs respectively of 113 and 111) and much of these differences seems likely to have been due to chance. The low relative risk in the participants from both chronic bronchitis and lung cancer suggests that participants may have smoked less than the controls and this is supported by the finding that the mortality from the other principal diseases related to smoking, but not from other diseases, was also lower in the participants. The relatively high mortality in the participants from 'other injury and poisoning' and the relatively low mortality from cancer of the kidney seem likely to be the chance findings that must be expected when so many different causes of death are examined.

The low mortality in both study groups from neoplasms and other non-violent causes of death compared with that expected from national mortality rates is largely explained by the fact that both groups contained a high proportion of Officers and men whose occupations would be classified in social class I by the Office of Population Censuses and Surveys, particularly in the older age groups in which most deaths occurred, and that both groups were highly selected for physical fitness.

Comparison of the mortality rates of the independent respondents who were respectively included in and omitted from the main study showed that the results were not substantially biased by the omission of some participants, but that the mortality rates observed might be slightly underestimated.

It is concluded that small hazards of leukaemia and multiple myeloma may well have been associated with participation in the nuclear weapons programme, but that their existence is certainly not proven. Participation has not otherwise had a detectable effect on the participants' expectation of life or on their total risk of developing cancer.

REFERENCES

[1] Darby, S. C., Kendall, G. M., Fell, T. P., O'Hagan, J. A., Muirhead, C. R., Ennis, J. R., Ball, A. M., Dennis, J. A., Doll, R. (1988) Mortality and Cancer Incidence in UK Participants in UK Atmospheric Nuclear Weapon Tests and Experimental Programmes. NRPB-R214.

[2] Darby, S. C., Kendall, G. M. Fell, T. P., O'Hagan, J. A., Muirhead, C. R., Ennis, J. A., Ball, A. M., Dennis, J. A., Doll, R. (1988) A summary of mortality and incidence of cancer in men from the United Kingdom who participated in the United Kingdom's atmospheric nuclear weapon tests and experimental programmes. Brit Med J, 296, 332-338.

THE TEST OF HYPOTHESIS AND LEUKAEMIA NEAR NUCLEAR INSTALLATIONS

R. Wakeford and K. Binks
(British Nuclear Fuels plc, Warrington, Cheshire)

and

D. Wilkie
(UK Atomic Energy Authority, Seascale, Cumbria)

ABSTRACT

The past decade has witnessed a burgeoning of interest in the levels of childhood leukaemia risk in areas near nuclear establishments. This interest has grown from media reports of excess cases of leukaemia occurring amongst children living in the vicinity of certain installations, and much epidemiological research work investigating these claims has ensued. These investigations have not been easy: childhood leukaemia has a low rate of incidence, generating small expected numbers which lead to low statistical power; only a few aetiological factors have been positively identified - the major causal factors (i.e. the main potential confounding factors) remain unknown; and there are difficulties arising from the quality of the available data. The distinction between a hypothesis-generating study and a hypothesis-testing study must remain clear if inferential problems are to be avoided. A critical review of the studies carried out so far reveals that several of the epidemiological investigations have suffered from various difficulties that render the interpretation of results unclear. Nevertheless, evidence does exist for elevated rates of childhood leukaemia incidence around (certain) nuclear installations. The reasons for this are uncertain, primarily due to a lack of understanding of the background distribution of childhood leukaemia cases, and of basic aetiology.

1. INTRODUCTION

> "The epidemiologist has to apply intellectual rigour to interpretating weak data, and his motto could well be 'dirty hands, but a clean mind' *(manus sordidae, mens pura)*."
>
> G. Rose and D.J.P. Barker [51,p14]

During the 1980s, considerable public concern and scientific debate have arisen out of various reports that the numbers of cases of childhood leukaemia which have occurred in areas near certain nuclear installations are greater than would be expected from national or regional rates of incidence. This subject has received much media attention, and television documentaries have been particularly prominent in publicising claims of unusual patterns of childhood leukaemia incidence in the neighbourhood of nuclear sites. The Government has responded by establishing initially the Independent Advisory Group in 1983, to specifically examine claims involving the Sellafield establishment in Cumbria, and then the Committee on Medical Aspects of Radiation in the Environment (COMARE) in 1985, to look into the whole question of health effects that might be due to environmental radioactivity.

Particular interest has focused upon the potential link between radioactive effluent and the reported case excesses. Radiological assessments carried out by the National Radiological Protection Board (NRPB) have persistently demonstrated [55], [74] that radiation doses from radioactive materials discharged from nuclear installations are far too low to account for any observed excesses of childhood leukaemia cases: almost invariably, these doses are much lower than the combination of natural, medical, fallout and other background sources of radiation. Nevertheless, COMARE has identified a number of speculative mechanisms whereby raised rates of incidence might be related to site operations, although not necessarily to site discharges (see Wheldon [72] for a good discussion).

The situation would appear to be: either,

1) the radiological protection community has remained ignorant of an important radiation risk factor which, alone or in combination with other factors, can produce a detectable excess of cases at existing levels of exposure; or
2) the reported excesses reflect genuinely raised risks of childhood leukaemia, but that these have no direct link with site operations involving radioactivity; or
3) the underlying risk of childhood leukaemia around these nuclear installations is not elevated above the national norm; or
4) the reports are due to some combination of the above.

Clearly, epidemiology has an important role to play in distinguishing between these possibilities; but the various problems involved with carrying out epidemiological studies in this area of work certainly demand Rose and Barker's "intellectual rigour" if a number of pitfalls are to be avoided. This is particularly so when continuing media interest ensures that these studies are conducted under a certain degree of pressure.

In this paper we shall examine the difficulties that are associated with the epidemiological investigation of childhood leukaemia incidence around nuclear installations. The frequency of occurrence and the current medical understanding of childhood leukaemia, and how these affect the available data and their treatment, are outlined, and the various shortcomings of the data are discussed. Then we examine how study formulation and design - in particular, the distinction between a hypothesis-generating and a hypothesis-testing study - have a crucial influence upon the interpretation of results. Next, we critically review the epidemiological studies of childhood leukaemia incidence and/or mortality around nuclear establishments that have been reported so far, paying particular attention to those features of a study which are examined earlier in the paper. Finally, as a result of this review, we make some concluding remarks.

2. BASIC EPIDEMIOLOGICAL CONSIDERATIONS

2.1 Power, Confounding and Data Bias

Those embarking upon epidemiological studies of childhood leukaemia incidence are confronted with a number of problems associated either with the fundamental nature and our present state of knowledge of leukaemia, or with the quality of the data to be employed within the analysis. In this subsection, we shall examine these problems.

Linet [47] states (p256):

> "It is clear that leukemias consist of several diverse, etiologically distinct diseases".

The pattern of leukaemia types suffered by children differs from that of adults, which probably indicates different risk factors [47]. The commonest type of leukaemia occurring in children (usually defined as persons under 15 years of age) is acute lymphoblastic leukaemia (ALL) which accounts for around 80% of childhood leukaemia cases in Britain [59]. A number of ALL subtypes have been identified, and some of these subtypes are closely related biologically to certain subtypes of childhood non-Hodgkin's lymphoma (NHL), which sometimes leads to difficulties in distinguishing between ALL and NHL [9, p79]. The annual rate of incidence of childhood ALL in Britain is low at around 27 cases per million children, the occurrence being most frequent in the 0-4 year age range and amongst boys [59].

Survival has improved from the position before 1960, when childhood leukaemia was almost invariably fatal, to the situation now, when treatment ensures that more than half of childhood ALL patients survive the disease. However, the biological basis for this treatment success is not understood [22]. Linet [47] states (p.260):

> "Despite great advances in many scientific disciplines in which in-depth study has focused upon leukemia pathogenesis and etiology, the risk factors identified account for only a small proportion of each of the leukemias."

The designers of epidemiological studies of childhood leukaemia are faced, therefore, with two major methodological difficulties:

(1) a low "background" incidence rate which produces small expected numbers of cases unless large populations and long time periods are involved; and

(2) unknown individual risk factors which may vary to an unknown extent both within and between populations.

The consequence of (1) is that small expected numbers lead to low statistical power, so that relatively large excess risks may go undetected because the aetiological factor under study has only a limited opportunity to express itself as observed cases, which can produce "false-negative" study results. The consequence of (2) is that, since inferences must be drawn from the statistical analysis of observational (rather than experimental) data, confounding by risk factors which correlate with the factor under investigation - and which operate in an uncontrolled manner within the population under study - can produce "false-positive" study results.

In general, statistical power will be enhanced by increasing the number of person-years under study. However, if persons or time periods irrelevant to the factor under study are included in the analysis, then this will reduce the power because of dilution of the excess risk within the study population. In addition, power will invariably be diminished by population migration: out-migration during the cancer latent period loses "exposed" cases from the area, and in-migration adds "unexposed" persons. Families with young children would appear to be particularly mobile [24], so migration effects could produce "false-negative" results in geographical studies of childhood cancer indicence based on home address at diagnosis, especially if small areas are involved [19].

The potentially distorting effects of confounding factors are usually dealt with either through the direct adjustment of expected numbers to account for the presence of such factors within the study population (for example, the age-sex structure), or through the comparison with a control population which has been "matched" for modifying factors (such as urban/rural status) with the population under investigation. However, such methods for dealing with confounding may only be of limited success when major risk factors - and hence major confounding factors - are not known with any certainty. Even if competing aetiological factors do not introduce bias into a study, their presence will inevitably inflate the variance of the observed distribution, and hence reduce the statistical power of the analysis [16].

Quite apart from the intrinsic methodological problems associated with the epidemiological study of childhood leukaemia is the question of data quality. The substantial rise in the childhood leukaemia survival rate which has occurred since 1960, should imply that incidence data will be preferable to mortality data. The use of incidence rather than mortality data will, in general, produce larger expected numbers, and also will avoid the introduction of bias and loss of power due to non-uniformity of treatment success and to migration in the period between diagnosis and death. However, cancer registration data are of variable quality [60] which leads to difficulties in interpreting raised registration rates. Cook-Mozaffari *et al.* [12] found that cancer registration efficiency has been especially high in areas near nuclear installations, and, as a consequence, Forman *et al.* [27] have used mortality data only in their analysis to avoid results which are artefacts of registration completeness.

A special search for cases in an area of particular interest will compound the problem of registration variability since this practice is liable to preferentially raise the completeness of the data in that area. Clearly, inaccurate case details (such as date of, or address at, diagnosis) could also introduce bias into and will reduce the sensitivity of - a study.

The decennial national census provides the basis of population estimates in population-based studies. Various methods may be employed to deal with population changes in the intercensal years (eg [12, p35]). Failure to deal adequately with population movements can lead to biased expected numbers because an erroneous "population at risk" is being employed. Such effects might be anticipated to be particularly disruptive if small areal units are being considered in a district where large-scale population movements have occurred (as a result, for example, of inner-city clearance).

Finally, the recorded numbers of childhood leukaemia cases may be affected by variations in diagnostic criteria. Diagnostic techniques have improved considerably over the years, and this introduces a possible source of bias into an analysis through temporal and geographical non-uniformity of disease identification and classification. Not only are leukaemia types and subtypes affected by these variations, but a problem of differentiating between ALL and NHL also exists - COMARE [9] has identified 3 cases of childhood NHL in or around Thurso which should be more appropriately classified as ALL. It is of interest that the latest of these cases was diagnosed in 1986, so classification problems are still to be found in some areas.

2.2 Hypothesis-Generation and Hypothesis-Testing

An underlying random selection process is capable of producing unusual groupings of events because chance alone will produce extreme deviations from an expected number, given sufficient opportunity [69]. Thus, even if the "background" risk of childhood leukaemia is independent of both time and space, noticeable "clusters" of cases may arise, purely by chance. Clearly, such random fluctuations in the background "noise" of disease incidence do not indicate locally raised risks. On the other hand, an elevated incidence rate could be the product of some factor which is operating to increase the risk of the disease of interest in that particular area. The retrospective identification of case excesses does not, in general, allow the genuine causal signal to be distinguished from the random background noise (see the reviews of Enterine [25] and Thomas [62]). As a consequence, the aetiological significance of the numerous reports of *a posteriori* "clusters" which have appeared in the literature over the years - such as the excess of multiple myeloma cases in the town of Thief River Falls, Minnesota ($O/E = 6/0.23$, $p = 10^{-7}$) [46], or of the 4 leukaemia cases associated with a single house in the southern USA [48] - is unclear [53]. There are, however, occasional instances where the Poisson probabilities generated are so remote that the observation can be judged *per se* to be the product of a large excess risk or of some data peculiarity. For example, in the City of London between 1969 and 1973, 18 deaths from leukaemia were recorded whereas only 1.24 deaths would be expected ($p<10^{-15}$) [49].

The difficulties of interpretation of case "clusters" are aggravated by the *post hoc* tightening of analysis boundaries (space, time, age, disease-type) around particular cases to make the grouping appear even more unusual. In 1968, Glass *et al* [34] drew attention to the fallacy of such action. They observed (p101):

"In the study of a relatively rare disease such as leukemia, it is important to keep in mind the possibility that seemingly high concentrations of cases may be generated by overzealous statistical manipulation."

It is clear that "overzealous statistical manipulation" of randomly distributed data can produce apparently impressive excesses over expectation, which have no bearing whatsoever upon the nature of the underlying "risk".

The effects of chance fluctuations may be quantified in a hypothesis-testing study. The interesting patterns observed in exploratory surveys of data should be used to generate hypotheses concerning the possible causal factors underlying the production of these patterns. These hypotheses may then be tested using relevant datasets which are independent of the data which generated the hypotheses. Smith and Pike [54] have emphasised this point (p660):

"Anecdotal reports may be of enormous value in the generation of hypotheses but, once this stage is past, such reports are usually of no value and may even be counterproductive of a proper test of the generated hypothesis."

Not only must the data employed within a hypothesis-testing study be independent of the data in the hypothesis-generating study, but the structure of the confirmatory study must not be influenced by knowledge of details of cases to be used in the study - the test of hypothesis must be set up "blind" of the study data. Any selection of dataset or analysis boundary which is influenced by prior knowledge is liable to bias the study results, because the analysis structure will not have accounted for such selection [16]. Selection bias means that, even if the background distribution of cases is random, the cumulative Poisson probability does not represent the "true" statistical significance of the resultant incidence ratio (O/E): the particular ratio is likely to have been chosen from the extremes of the observed distribution, and the unadjusted Poisson probability $P(\geq O|E)$ is no longer a legitimate measure of statistical significance under these circumstances. Davies and Inskip [19] strongly endorse this principle of "blind" hypothesis-testing (p9):

"It cannot be emphasised too strongly that when testing a hypothesis there can be no exploration: the precise comparisons to be made must be defined in advance without prior knowledge of the results. To look first at the results, and then to choose the district, age-group and date definitions which most stongly support the hypothesis (or most strongly refute it) constitutes manipulation of the data with hindsight, and is a form of scientific dishonesty."

If a hypothesis-testing study has been set up correctly, then the probability that a chance deviation from the assumed expected value has produced the observed result is known. Thus, the effects of random fluctuations under the statistical model of the null hypothesis (the hypothesis of "no effect" from factors other than those accounted for in generating the expected number) are quantified. The investigator employs a preselected significance level, α, to reject the null hypothesis if the cumulative probability associated with the study result is less than α, and thereby accepts that the null hypothesis will produce a "false-positive" result (a "type I error") with a probability of α. A hypothesis-testing study with high statistical power can allow the adoption of a small value of α, which reduces the risk of such an error. However, the insidious presence of confounding factors must always be borne in mind.

The problem of type I errors is intensified when multiple comparisons are carried out within a study. In the simplest case of n independent, continuous-distribution significance tests being performed, each with a significance level set to α, the probability γ of finding at least one result significant at the α level by chance alone is

$$\gamma = 1 - (1 - \alpha)^n.$$

Therefore, if the overall type I error rate γ in the study is to be reduced to an acceptable value, then each individual significance level should be set to

$$\alpha = 1 - (1 - \gamma)^{1/n} \approx \gamma/n,$$

the Bonferroni limit [43]. However, unless the individual significance tests have high statistical power, this strategy can lead to the opposite problem of "false-negative" results ("type II errors") because of the stringent significance levels employed. Such difficulties can be reduced in a hypothesis-testing study by clearly identifying at the design stage of the study the specific *a priori* hypotheses under test, and (when data permit) by making significance tests as powerful as possible so that small α values may be employed. However, during data exploration significance tests must be applied with care, and with the aim of identifying interesting associations which should then be the subject of studies designed to test the validity of the potential relationships [12].

The investigator must be particularly guarded over the interpretation of data patterns which have been identified without the use of a preselected analysis framework. *Post hoc* boundaries used to describe such case groupings are only one particular set out of a large, and generally unquantifiable, number of possible (non-independent) sets of boundaries. The meaning of such results cannot be properly assessed without a subsequent confirmatory study using independent data, because of this problem of multiplicity. This is the reason for the warning of Glass *et al.* [34] concerning "overzealous statistical manipulation".

3. THE STUDIES SO FAR

In this section we shall examine the studies of childhood leukaemia incidence and/or mortality around nuclear installations that have been carried out so far, paying particular attention to those aspects of epidemiology which are considered in the previous section.

3.1 Sellafield

On 1 November 1983, a Yorkshire Television (YTV) documentary entitled "Windscale - the Nuclear Laundry" (producer, Mr. J.A. Cutler) was broadcast throughout the United Kingdom. The programme claimed that YTV researchers had found an unusually large number of leukaemia and other cancer cases in the population of young people living to the south of the British Nuclear Fuels plc (BNFL) Sellafield nuclear establishment (which includes, amongst other facilities, the Windscale irradiated nuclear fuel reprocessing plants and the Calder Hall Magnox nuclear reactors), situated on the West Cumbrian coast. In particular, the programme claimed that the incidence of leukaemias in the young children (0-9 years of age) of the nearby coastal village of Seascale was especially unusual: for the period 1956-80, "$O = 5$, $E = 0.45$, $p<0.0002$", [66]. Owing to the possible link between an excess of childhood cancer cases and radioactive effluent discharges, the documentary triggered intense interest in the news media. After the programme had been shown, the Minister of Health asked Sir Douglas Black to head an independent inquiry to examine the claims that had been made. The report of this inquiry, the "Black Report", was published in July 1984, some nine months after the broadcast of the documentary [40].

The Black Group was faced with a number of difficulties of interpretation of the epidemiological evidence presented by the television team. The Black Report notes [40, p11, para 2.2]

> "Mr. Cutler, the producer of the YTV film, told us that his original intention had been to look at the effects of occupational exposure to radiation in the nuclear power industry, and that initially he had approached BNFL

> at Sellafield with this in mind .... . However, the attention of the YTV team was drawn to a number of children with leukaemia in Seascale. This led them to change the direction of their investigation, and to concentrate on the general population living near Sellafield".

The television team did not, therefore, carry out an investigation of childhood leukaemia incidence in Seascale with the preconceived notion that these were the diseases and the place that should be examined if the health effects of radioactive discharges were to be observed, but made a serendipitous discovery of the excess of cases through anecdotal reports once they were in the locality. This led to the principal problem of interpretation of the data for the Black Group: knowing that extreme variations of disease rates can occur by chance alone, how can a decision be confidently reached as to whether the Seascale childhood leukaemia incidence rate represents a genuinely raised risk in the village or not? This question is not just confined to small area fluctuations in the rate of incidence of childhood leukaemia, but extends to other age groups and disease types that might have been considered as equally worthy of attention by a television producer. For example, on 27 April 1983, another television documentary "Dying for Action" was broadcast, which claimed, among other things, that an unusually large number of multiple myeloma cases had occurred amongst the adults of Barrow-in-Furness, Cumbria [42], and the programme highlighted Sellafield radioactive discharges as a potential cause. Clearly, a large, but unquantifiable, number of choices were potentially available to Mr. Cutler before viewing the data.

Hutchison has argued [39, p11]

> "If you were asked to predict likely areas for an excess of radiation related illnesses, would you or would you not go for that around Sellafield, with a record of discharging quantities of radioactive materials roughly one hundred times as great as all the rest of Britain's nuclear plants put together (Black Report Figure 1.1). If it was going to be anywhere, it would be there. A priori rules ok?"

Although this argument is superficially attractive, it does not address the central questions as to which "radiation related illnesses" and what "area around Sellafield" would have been selected in advance of inspecting the data. One may employ this sort of reasoning to arrive at some qualitative judgement as to whether the Seascale childhood leukaemia cases should be the subject of further study, but it will not allow a quantitative assessment of statistical significance because the answers are only legitimate if they are not influenced by a knowledge of the available data.

Having received hearsay evidence concerning childhood cancer incidence in Seascale, the YTV team set about collecting details of cancer cases which had occurred in the vicinity of Sellafield. The television researchers did not have access to medically confidential information, so unconventional methods were used, such as the interviewing of local inhabitants, to obtain these details. Care is required in handling data collected in this manner because, quite apart from the possibility of erroneous information, special searches for cases are liable to yield data that are more complete for the area of interest than for comparison areas. This could lead to an artificially high incidence ratio.

Having collected data in this way, the YTV researchers collated the information as mortality and incidence rates. Figure 1 shows how these rates were presented [17]. The figure provides a good illustration of boundary tightening around known cases: age groups, cancer types and geographical areas have been selected according to observed case details, and the sole raison d'etre for the "five coastal parishes" as a study unit would appear to be the presence of the cancer cases contained within their boundaries. In addition, the Millom RD and "five coastal parishes" rates are for the period 1963-80, whilst the Seascale rate is for the period 1956-80, to include two cases which occurred during the period 1956-1962 [66]. Furthermore, it will be noted from Figure 1 that rates for Ennerdale RD, which includes Sellafield and the coastal area to the north have not been presented, even though this district might have been considered to be of as much interest, *a priori* as Millom RD. However, it would appear that the cancer rates for Ennerdale RD are not particularly unusual [40].

The one area to the north of Sellafield which has been the subject of media attention is Maryport, a town some 40 km along the coast from Sellafield. Another YTV documentary "Return to Windscale" (producer, Mr. J.A. Cutler), broadcast on 3 April 1984, claimed that the cancer mortality rate during the second half of 1963-82 for 15-24 years olds living in Maryport was unusually high [66]. However, the rate was generated using suspiciously tight time and age boundaries, and Maryport would also appear to have been singled out from a district possessing a generally low cancer mortality rate for this time period and age group [40]. It is quite possible that this highlighted rate is simply an artefact of boundary tightening. Once again, the difficulties of interpretation that result from the selection of boundaries *ex post facto* are apparent.

The Black Group was able to confirm that the epidemiological data for Millom RD gathered by the YTV team were, in general, accurate. However, the problem of *post hoc* boundaries was not so easy to address. Apart from determining that West Cumbrian cancer rates were generally at expected levels, the Black Report did not attempt to deal comprehensively with the post-data selection of age groups and disease types; but the Report did try to assess the influence that the choice of geographical areas and time periods might have had upon the results of the YTV analysis. A number of studies, based upon routinely collected data and employing conventional analysis boundaries, were carried out on behalf of the Black Group. Three of these studies used geographical units which were sufficiently small to allow the YTV results to be directly compared.

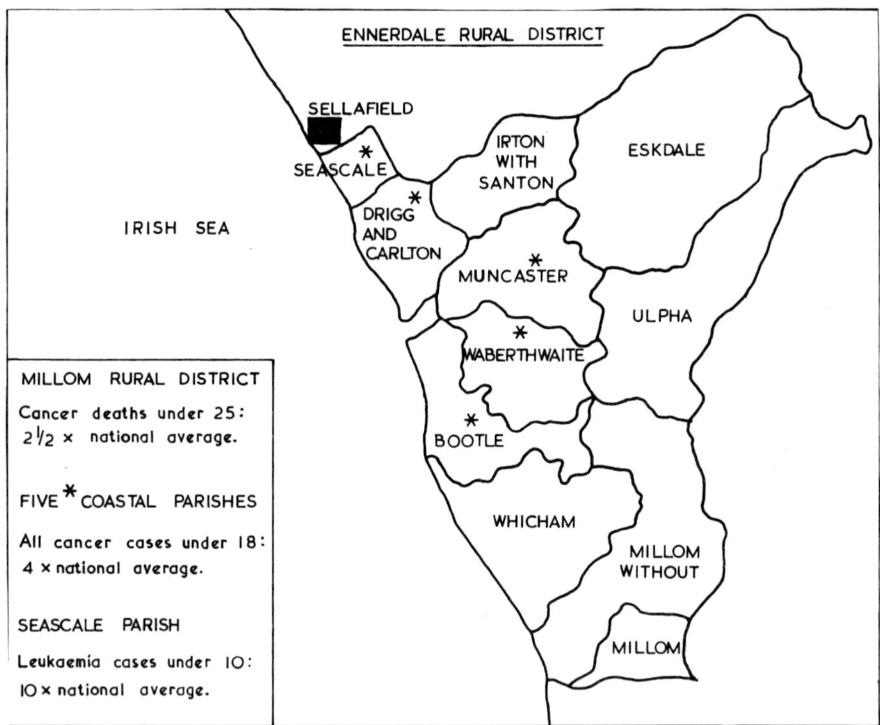

Fig. 1 The 11 parishes of pre-1974 Millom Rural District to the south of Sellafield, and the geographical, age and disease boundaries employed by the Yorkshire Television researchers to generate the mortality and incidence rates used in the television documentary [17].

1. Gardner and Winter [33] examined 0-24 year old leukaemia mortality ratios for the 14 pre-1974 local authority areas of the pre-1974 county of Cumberland, for the two time periods 1959-67 and 1968-78. Millom RD during 1968-78 had the mortality ratio (O/E = 6/1.4) with the lowest one-tailed Poisson probability (p = 0.003) of the 28 ratios under study. However, had the 0-14 year age range - which is the conventional age range used for the study of childhood leukaemia [22] - been used, then the ratio for Wigton RD (in northern Cumberland) during 1959-67 (O/E = 6/1.6) would have possessed the lowest p (= 0.006, cf.p = 0.07 for the 1968-78 Millom RD childhood leukaemia ratio of O/E = 3/0.95).

2. Gardner and Winter extended their study of under 25 year old leukaemia mortality ratios during 1968-78, to 151 Rural Districts in England and Wales of similar size to Millom RD [40]. Of the 152 ratios under study, Millom RD had the second highest, the highest being for Depwade RD in Norfolk (O/E = 8/1.8, p = 0.0006) [29].

3. Craft *et al.* [14] examined childhood (0-14 years of age) "lymphoid malignancy" (ALL and the lymphomas) incidence in the 675 electoral wards of the Northern Health Region of England during 1968-82. Seascale ward (which corresponds to Seascale parish as used by the YTV researchers) had the incidence ratio (O/E = 4/0.25) with the lowest one-tailed Poisson probability (p = 0.0001), although no other ward in the vicinity of Sellafield possessed an unusual incidence rate.

From these studies, the Black Report concluded [40, p33, para 2.40]:

> "The Seascale incidence and Millom Rural District mortality rates for leukaemia among young people are unusual, though not unparalleled".

Thus, from the epidemiological evidence presented to them, the Black Group was able to confirm that an unusually large number of leukaemia cases or deaths had occurred in the young people living to the south of Sellafield, but given the circumstances surrounding the discovery of these cases or deaths, the excess was not sufficiently large for a non-random effect to be inferred *per se*. The Black Report could not (and could not be expected to) distinguish between the excess being the signal of some aetiological factor operating in the area and a chance sampling fluctuation about a spatially uniform underlying risk. The Report notes that the fact that other electoral wards or Rural Districts with increased rates are geographically scattered outside the area around Sellafield may indicate that this excess is not due to some factor unique to the Sellafield area. In addition, Hargreaves *et al.* [35] have pointed out that the geographical and temporal patterns of incidence of leukaemias and lymphomas within Millom RD are not what might have been predicted if radioactive discharges were to be responsible for the excess cases.

Since the radiological evidence [58] which was provided to the Black Group could not explain the excess of childhood leukaemia cases in Seascale in terms of radiation exposure due to radionuclides discharged with the Sellafield effluent (the difference between observed and predicted numbers being a factor of at least 400), the Black Report considered that the case for a causal link between these childhood leukaemia cases and Sellafield operations was "not proven", and offered a "qualified reassurance" to those concerned about health effects in the neighbourhood of Sellafield. However, it was recognised that "unavoidable uncertainties" existed in the assessment of the risk of radiation-induced leukaemia, including the possibility that some unrecognised pathway of exposure existed. The Report made ten recommendations, mostly for further epidemiological and radiological work to improve understanding of the risk of childhood leukaemia in the Sellafield area, and all these recommendations were accepted by the Government. It was clearly correct to investigate the possible causes of the excess cases further. As Cuzick has observed of the "cluster" of childhood leukaemia cases near Sellafield [18]:

> "If it [the 'cluster'] occurred at some non-specific location, such a cluster would almost certainly be dismissed as chance, but its proximity to a source of exposure to a substance known to cause leukaemia changes the context of observation".

This seems to be an entirely reasonable and scientific position to adopt under these circumstances.

However, those involved with the original YTV investigation were dissatisfied with the cautious conclusions of the Black Report. Urquhart and Cutler [64] noted that they had identified several West Cumbrian cases which had been omitted from the epidemiological studies used by the Black Group in their investigation, and also suggested that if all childhood malignancies (rather than just the leukaemias and lymphomas) were considered, then the unusual geographical pattern of incidence extends beyond just Seascale. In particular, they drew attention to the geographical distribution of the 10 (out of a total of 675) wards in the Northern Region with childhood cancer incidence ratios for 1968-82 possessing the lowest associated one-tailed Poisson probabilities [15, p54, Table 1]:

"Of the first ten wards [with the lowest probabilities] four are from the West Coast of Cumbria, and since that area has only thirty-seven wards adjoining the coast or tidal estuaries ... the probability of getting these four significant wards near the Cumbrian coast by chance is less than 1 in 700" [64].

However, a number of points must be considered:

(i) one of these 4 wards (Bootle) is only included in the first 10 because missing cases have been added, and this may have biased results due to preferential treatment of an area of interest.

(ii) The 37 coastal or estuarine wards are neither from Cumbria as a whole, nor from just West Cumbria, but this grouping does provide rather tight boundaries around the northernmost and southernmost wards (Wampool and Barrow Island respectively) of the 4 Cumbrian wards of interest.

(iii) It is debatable whether Wampool ward (an inland area surrounding Wigton) [15, p56, Figure 3] would have been classified as coastal or estuarine prior viewing results.

So, as with the original study of the YTV team, it is difficult to interpret the results of Urquhart and Cutler [64] because of the *post hoc* analysis structure.

The Committee on Medical Aspects of Radiation in the Environment (COMARE) was established in 1985 as a result of a recommendation in the Black Report. In 1986, COMARE made a detailed re-examination of Sellafield discharges, particularly the accidental releases of the 1950s and early 1960s, and found that the estimates of discharged material would have to be revised upwards [8]. However, as the radiological assessment for the Black Report had been based, whenever possible, upon environmental monitoring results rather than discharge records, the predicted number of radiation-induced childhood leukaemia cases in Seascale was increased by a factor of less than 2, leaving a discrepancy between observed and predicted numbers of at least a factor of 250 [56],[57]. COMARE concluded [8, p22]:

"Taking the evidence presented in the Black Advisory Group Report, there is an apparent excess incidence of leukaemia in Seascale and there continue to be four possible explanations for this apparent excess:

a. it is due to chance;

b it is due to exposure to environmental radiation;

c it is due to a high sensitivity to leukaemia induction of members of the population of Seascale (we know of no evidence for this and in view of the mobile nature of this population this seems unlikely);

d. it is due to some as yet undetected environmental agent such as a chemical or virus.

It is quite likely that the excess was caused by some combination of two or more of the above factors".

Some of the epidemiological studies recommended by the Black Report have now been completed. Gardner *et al.* [31], [32] studied cancer incidence amongst the Seascale birth cohort (those born during 1950-83 to a mother resident in the village) and amongst the schools cohort (those born since 1950 to a mother resident outside the village, but attending a school in Seascale before the end of 1984). They were able to confirm the excess of cancer cases (O=12, E=2.8), particularly childhood leukaemia cases (O=6, E=0.6) and childhood NHL cases (O=2), in the birth cohort, but found no excess in the schools cohort. This pattern of incidence might have been anticipated from the data presented in the Black Report, but the cohort studies were able to demonstrate that the high childhood leukaemia incidence rate for Seascale found by the Black Group was not just an artificial product of inaccuracies in expected numbers due to population movements. Although the cohort studies data are not independent of the data used in the Black Report - only one further case of childhood leukaemia was discovered in those who had left Seascale - Gardner *et al.* speculated that the difference between the results for the two cohorts could be due to some factor operating before, or soon after, birth. Gardner is also directing a case-control study of leukaemia and lymphoma cases which have occurred in West Cumbria since 1950. This study will examine the possible influence of a number of factors upon the incidence of these diseases in West Cumbria, and should generate a number of hypotheses for testing in subsequent studies.

Bithell and Stone [6] have developed a statistical method that selects the maximum incidence or mortality ratio from those ratios associated with all the practicably possible cumulative distance zones around a source of putative risk, and then determines the statistical significance of obtaining this maximum ratio under the assumption of a uniform risk, taking account of the process of selection. One of the advantages of this "Poisson maximum test" is that it tackles the problem of the *post hoc* selection of the geographical area used in an analysis. Bithell and Stone have applied this test to the 1968-82 childhood leukaemia incidence data for the electoral wards of Cumbria, obtained from the database of Craft *et al.* [15], with cumulative distance zones constructed from wards ranked by distance from Sellafield, treated as a point source of risk. As might be anticipated from the study of Craft *et al.* [15], the innermost distance zone (corresponding to Seascale ward [6]) possesses the maximum incidence ratio, and in this situation the significance of the Poisson maximum statistic will be almost the same as the cumulative Poisson probability for the Seascale ward ratio (ie. p<0.0001) [6]. However, Bithell and Stone remark that once the 4 Seascale cases are removed from the analysis, there is very little evidence of any locational association of childhood leukaemia incidence with Sellafield. This analysis confirms the remoteness of finding a childhood leukaemia incidence ratio as large as that observed at Seascale, this near to Sellafield. However, the test does not address the *post hoc* selection of either childhood leukaemia as the health effect, or Sellafield as the location, used in the analysis. The "maximum Poisson test" would be of value in testing the hypothesis generated by the initial Sellafield observations around other nuclear installations, and Wakeford *et al.* [70] have carried out a similar type of analysis around Dounreay (see the next subsection).

Following concern in Ireland over the possible health effects of radioactive discharges from Sellafield into the Irish Sea, in March 1985 the UK Government established the Independent Committee (chaired by Professor W.S.B. Lowry) to examine patterns of disease in Northern Ireland for any features which might be due to radiation exposure. The Lowry Committee examined, amongst other health effects, childhood (0-14 years of age) leukaemia incidence and mortality in Northern Ireland, and the results of the study were published in the Final Report of the Committee in 1989 [41]. The Committee found that cancer registration data were not of a sufficiently high quality to be the sole source of data for the childhood leukaemia incidence study, and information from other sources (such as hospital records) was also employed. For the childhood leukaemia studies, the Committee classified the 526 electoral wards of the Province as either coastal (135 wards) or inland, and examined two time periods (1968-76 and 1977-85), although only the latter period was used for the incidence study because of doubts over the completeness of the earlier data. The incidence ratio for the coastal division (O/E = 39/36.4) was not significantly different from that of the inland division (O/E = 114/116.6). The mortality ratios for the coastal division (1968-76 O/E = 22/21.4; 1977-85 O/E = 15/19.3) were not significantly different from those of the inland division (1968-76 O/E = 80/74.6; 1977-85 O/E = 60/61.6). As a consequence, the Committee concluded that Sellafield discharges had no discernible influence upon the risk of childhood leukaemia in the coastal division of Northern Ireland during 1968-85.

It is of interest (and perhaps surprising) that neither the Black Report nor the 1986 COMARE Report made explicit mention of the possibility of conducting hypothesis-testing studies of childhood leukaemia incidence around other nuclear installations in Britain (or elsewhere), using the exploratory West Cumbrian observations to generate suitable hypotheses. It could be that since the Sellafield radioactive discharges are both quantitatively and qualitatively somewhat unique (as we have seen Hutchison remark [39]), it was not thought that such studies would prove to be particularly helpful in the investigation of an effect which may be more or less confined to the Sellafield area. In any case, the low power generally associated with these studies would lead to problems in interpreting "negative" results: for example, for a true relative risk of 1.5 and an expected number of 10, a one-sided Poisson test with a significance level set at 0.05 has a power of less than 50%. Nevertheless, a number of studies of childhood leukaemia incidence and/or mortality around other nuclear establishments have been carried out since the publication of the Black Report; but, with the exception of the studies of Cook-Mozaffari *et al.* [12], [13], the piecemeal nature of these investigations has generated inferential difficulties, in that the reasons either for certain analyses being carried out, or for the adoption of certain boundaries within an analysis, are unclear.

3.2 Scottish Installations, Particularly Dounreay

Heasman *et al.* [36] submitted evidence on young leukaemia incidence around the Scottish nuclear installations at Hunterston, Chapelcross and Dounreay during 1968-81, to the Black Advisory Group. No especially unusual results were reported, apart from a raised incidence rate for the Hunterston area in the second half of the time period (O/E = 18/9.13, p = 0.006).

In 1986, Heasman *et al.* published the results of a further analysis of young leukaemia and lymphoma incidence in the Dounreay area during 1968-84 [37]. This analysis was carried out for a public local inquiry into plans to expand operations at the Dounreay site. For the area within 12.5 km of Dounreay, a raised leukaemia incidence rate for the 0-24 year old age group during 1979-84 was reported (O/E = 5/0.513, p = 0.00015). This finding prompted an investigation by COMARE [9].

Unfortunately, the interpretation of this result is not straightforward, since both geographical and temporal boundaries appear to have been selected after inspection of the data [9], [69]: the 12.5 km radius circle transects Thurso (the only town near Dounreay) in such a way as to include the 4 cases which have occurred in the town during 1968-84 within the 12.5 km boundary, and the 1979-84 period contains the years of diagnosis of all the young leukaemia cases in the Dounreay area. We have examined the boundary selection difficulties at length elsewhere [69], and the COMARE Second Report [9, Section 4.3] provides a good discussion of the statistical issues involved. COMARE considers that an appropriate geographical area for the examination of leukaemia incidence would be the area lying within 25 km of Dounreay, and an appropriate time interval the full 1968-84 period. With these boundaries, the elevated incidence ratio is much less marked and not significant (O/E = 6/2.95, p = 0.079).

However, COMARE has noted that two cases of non-Hodgkin's lymphoma which had occurred within 25 km of Dounreay during 1968-84 should be more appropriately classified as acute lymphoblastic leukaemia. If the incidence of leukaemias plus non-Hodgkin's lymphomas are analysed, then the incidence ratio (O/E = 8/3.86, p = 0.039) is significantly elevated (0.05 level). In addition, Wakeford *et al.* [70] have conducted a simulation exercise with randomly distributed cases to determine the "true" significance of the result for the 12.5 km radius area and the 1979-84 interval: if radii and time periods (within the principal 25 km and 1968-84 boundaries) were to be chosen on the basis of the viewed (simulated) data so as to minimise the one-tailed Poisson probability p associated with a selected incidence ratio, then a ratio with $p \leq 0.00015$ will occur with a frequency of 1.37% (95% CI 1.30-1.44). This frequency is about two orders of magnitude greater than would be expected from a direct interpretation of a result with an associated p = 0.00015, ie. assuming an *a priori* analysis structure. Nevertheless, this frequency is significantly low (0.05 level).

Despite the inferential difficulties posed by the Dounreay study, COMARE concluded that [9, p93]:

> "the evidence of a raised incidence of leukaemia near Dounreay, taken in conjunction with that relating to the area around Sellafield, tends to support the hypothesis that some feature of the nuclear plants that we have examined leads to an increased risk of leukaemia in young people living in the vicinity of those plants".

However, a radiological assessment carried out by the NRPB concluded that the predicted number of young leukaemias caused by radioactive discharges was at least a factor of 1000 less than the observed number [20]. COMARE made a number of recommendations for further work in order that this common aetiological "feature", whether connected with radiation or otherwise, be identified as rapidly as possible. What is clear is that the cases in the Dounreay area lend themselves to a hypothesis-testing case-control study, using as preselected factors of interest the results from the West Cumbrian case-control study.

We have examined the results of studies of young leukaemia incidence in the neighbourhood of other Scottish nuclear installations in some detail elsewhere [69]. In summary, no clear indication of an excess risk was apparent from these studies.

3.3 *Aldermaston and Burghfield*

On 3 December 1985, the Yorkshire Television (YTV) documentary "Inside Britain's Bomb" (producer Mr. J.A. Cutler) was broadcast. This programme claimed that YTV researchers had found that during 1971-85 a greater than expected number of leukaemia and lymphoma cases had occurred amongst the young people resident in 9 electoral wards in the vicinity of the Ministry of Defence (MoD) nuclear weapons establishments at Aldermaston and Burghfield, situated some 8 km apart in West Berkshire. Urquhart *et al.* [65] have presented the results of the YTV investigation and these are summarised in Table 1. The only result of note is that for under 5 year old children living in the wards associated with MoD Burghfield.

Area	Numbers of observed (O) and expected (E) cases in each age group (years)					
	0-4		5-14		15-24	
	O	E	O	E	O	E
Aldermaston "circle" of wards	2	1.1	1	1.6	4	2.2
Burghfield "circle" of wards	5*	0.8	1	1.2	2	1.5

* $p < 0.01$

Table 1

Observed and expected numbers of leukaemia and lymphoma cases in three age groups, diagnosed whilst resident in electoral wards lying within approximately 4 km of the MoD establishments at Aldermaston and Burghfield during 1971-85. Expected numbers are generated from registration rates for England and Wales during 1976-81 and from 1971 and 1981 census data. Data from Urquhart *et al* [65].

Unfortunately, Urquhart *et al.* do not state how the two MoD establishments came to be selected for investigation, nor do they reveal how the group of 9 wards and the 1971-85 time interval were chosen. As with the YTV study in the Sellafield area, cases were ascertained through local inquiries made by a YTV researcher. It is also of note that 6 of the 8 leukaemia and lymphoma cases in the 5-24 year age group are cases of Hodgkin's disease [65], a type of lymphoma which had not been identified previously as being of particular interest in relation to nuclear establishments. The many uncertainties associated with the YTV investigation present serious difficulties to a meaningful interpretation of the findings.

After learning that the YTV documentary was about to be shown, Barton *et al.* [5] published preliminary findings from a study of under 10 year old leukaemia registrations in West Berkshire during 1972-84. Their results showed a significant excess of 0-4 year old registrations (O=34, E=20.6, $p<0.01$), but no excess in the 5-9 year age group (O=11, E = 12.7). However, the authors warned [5]:

> "The apparent statistical significance of the excess in children under 5 must be interpreted with caution because we were already suspicious that there was an excess in children and this was the reason for the analysis".

They also noted that variations in registration efficiency, and that factors such as socio-economic class, could artificially inflate the O/E ratio.

Roman *et al.* [50] have presented the final results of this study in an analysis of childhood leukaemia incidence in the West Berkshire and the neighbouring Basingstoke and North Hampshire District Health Authorities during 1972-85. They found a significant excess of 0-14 year old leukaemia registrations in electoral wards with over half their area lying within 10 km of either the Aldermaston or the Burghfield installation (or both) or the Harwell installation, when compared with an expected number based on national registration rates (O/E = 41/28.6, $p<0.05$). (The Harwell establishment is situated about 2 km outside the study area, and the contribution of Harwell to the incidence ratio is small, O/E = 0/0.39). The excess of childhood leukaemia cases is confined to the 0-4 year age group (O/E = 29/14.4, $p<0.001$), although there was no prior reason for predicting this particular age distribution. In addition, the case excess is dominated by registrations in the Burghfield circle of wards (O/E = 38/23.9, $p<0.05$), the ratio for the Aldermaston circle alone being unremarkable (O/E = 8/6.4). The difference between the expected numbers for the two circles of wards is largely due to the inclusion of the town of Reading within the Burghfield circle.

Roman *et al.* did not discern any temporal pattern in the incidence of childhood leukaemia in the study area, nor was there strong evidence of any trend of incidence ratio with distance from an installation. Incidence ratios for the group of wards lying outside the 10 km circles were non-significantly raised - O/E = 48/40.8 and 24/19.6 for the 0-14 year and 0-4 year age groups respectively - and the authors noted that there is no significant difference between the ratios for wards within the circles and those for wards lying outside. However, they also observed that this latter comparison has low statistical power.

Wakeford *et al.* [69] considered that the findings of Roman *et al.* must be treated cautiously because:

(i) suspicion of an excess of childhood leukaemia registrations was the reason for the analysis [5];
(ii) the results for the 0-4 year age subgroup were not obtained because of *a priori* interest in this age range;
(iii) childhood cancer registration efficiency may be particularly high in this area [68] (Barclay [2] has noted the variable completeness of childhood leukaemia registrations within the area covered by the Wessex Cancer Registry, which includes the Basingstoke and North Hampshire DHA - see Subsection 3.5.);
(iv) the excess is largely associated with the Burghfield facility, which has been excluded, *a priori*, from other studies (eg. [12]) because it discharges only negligible quantities of tritium [21], [28]. (In fact, the radiation doses due to discharges from Burghfield are likely to be less than those received from a number of industrial, medical and research establishments in Reading, which lies within the Burghfield 10 km circle [21]). Had the Burghfield circle of wards not been included in the study of Roman *et al.*, then the null hypothesis would not have been rejected.

COMARE has considered the evidence for an excess of childhood leukaemia cases around Aldermaston and Burghfield in the COMARE Third Report [10]. For this report, the Childhood Cancer Research Group (CCRG) examined the incidence of childhood cancers other than leukaemia during 1971-82 within the same sets of wards as employed by Roman *et al.* The CCRG study showed an elevated incidence ratio for the wards lying within the 10 km circles for the 0-14 year age group (O/E = 61/47.5, $p<0.05$), which was largely due to excess cases in the 0-4 year age group (O/E = 30/19.4, $p<0.05$). For the wards which lie outside the circles, non-significantly raised ratios were found (0-14 year: O/E = 82/68.2; 0-4 year: O/E = 33/26.3). The difference between the ratios for the two groups of wards is not significant. (The COMARE report did not state whether the case excesses found by CCRG were due to any particular type(s) of childhood cancer, or how the excess for wards within the circles was split between Aldermaston and Burghfield). Therefore, the pattern of results for childhood cancers other than leukaemia is very similar to that for childhood leukaemia. The excesses of childhood leukaemia cases found at Seascale and around Dounreay were not accompanied by excesses of childhood cancers other than leukaemia (with the possible exception of non-Hodgkin's lymphoma); but these "negative" results must be viewed cautiously because of the small expected numbers involved.

It is clear that raised registration rates for both childhood leukaemia and childhood cancers other than leukaemia exist in the area covered by the West Berkshire and the Basingstoke and North Hampshire District Health Authorities, when compared with national rates. However, there is no significant difference between the rates for the 10 km circles of wards around Aldermaston and Burghfield, and the rates for the group of remaining wards. The possibility must be considered that the Aldermaston and Burghfield "positive" result arose solely out of the selection of these establishments for study because of the prior suspicion that a raised childhood leukaemia registration rate existed in West Berkshire [5], whatever the reason for this raised rate might be, and the status of MoD Burghfield within the study of Roman *et al.* must be treated with particular caution.

A detailed radiological assessment carried out by the NRPB has confirmed the very low radiation doses resulting from discharges from Aldermaston and Burghfield [21]. For example, radiation-induced leukaemia risks due to peak annual doses received by 1 year old children at 5 km from the two installations due to discharges are, respectively, factors of 3.4×10^4 and 1.9×10^8 less than the risk due to the annual dose from natural background radiation. The radiation doses due to the discharges of nuclear material from Aldermaston have been calculated to be less than those due to radionuclides in the effluent of the coal-fired boilers at that site, and these, in turn, are less than the doses due to emissions from the nearby coal-fired power station at Didcot [71]. The NRPB assessment of the radiological impact of the discharges from Aldermaston and Burghfield concludes [21, p28]:

"In no way can they [the discharges] be responsible for an increased incidence of leukaemia amongst children, if such an increased incidence is shown to exist".

COMARE also concluded that the discharges had been [10, p31]:

"far too low to account for the observed increase in childhood cancer incidence in the area".

The COMARE Third Report [10] made a number of recommendations, prominent amongst which was the Committee's view that further investigations of claims of raised levels of childhood leukaemia incidence around individual nuclear installations would not be fruitful until the underlying pattern of incidence throughout the country was better understood. To this end, COMARE recommended that efforts be made to obtain a high quality childhood cancer incidence database for the whole of Britain, so that incidence rates in particular areas may be considered against the background distribution of cases. The availability of such a database would also allow the effects of the selection of study areas on the basis of prior knowledge of data to be properly assessed.

3.4 Harwell

The Atomic Energy Research Establishment at Harwell in Oxfordshire, is situated just to the north of the West Berkshire boundary, and two West Berkshire electoral wards did meet the criterion of Roman *et al.* for being considered to be geographically associated with Harwell [50]. However, as these two wards provided only limited information on the incidence of childhood leukaemia in the vicinity of Harwell (O = 0, E = 0.39), the Childhood Cancer Research Group (CCRG) examined childhood (0-14 years) leukaemia registrations during 1971-82 in the area consisting of all wards with over half their area lying within 10 km of Harwell [10]. No excess of cases was found (O=4, E=5.87), and the 95% confidence interval for the incidence ratio is 0.19-1.75. The incidence ratio for childhood cancers other than leukaemia is greater than unity, but not significantly so (O/E = 15/11.5). For the 0-4 year age group, the subgroup of most interest in the Aldermaston and Burghfield study [50], incidence ratios were unremarkable for both leukaemias and other cancers (O/E = 3/3.05 and O/E = 5/4.75 respectively). The "negative" results for Harwell contrast with the "positive" results for Aldermaston and Burghfield, particularly because assessed radiation doses in the vicinity of Harwell, although at least three orders of magnitude lower than the doses received from natural background radiation, are higher than those in the vicinity of the MoD establishments [21]. A relatively small expected number (E = 5.87) makes the interpretation of the childhood leukaemia incidence ratio of 0.68 rather difficult; but the result is of interest because the CCRG study was not prompted by a prior suspicion of a raised incidence rate.

3.5 Winfrith

Barclay [3] has carried out a descriptive study of the incidence of childhood (0-15 years of age rather than the more usual 0-14 years of age) acute lymphoblastic leukaemia in Wessex during 1972-83, and especially in Dorset during 1972-85, in response to claims that excess cases had occurred in the neighbourhood of the Atomic Energy Establishment at Winfrith, Dorset. The study examined a number of aspects of the geographical distribution of cases, including a claim that living in cul-de-sacs or near water hydrants or valves was associated with childhood ALL incidence!

The search for cases which had occurred in Dorset and certain other districts of Wessex went beyond the local cancer registry (the Wessex Cancer Registry), and it is of interest that the use of sources such as haematology department notes revealed that only 80% of the Dorset childhood ALL cases were registered on the Wessex Cancer Registry.

Barclay observed that 3 cases of childhood ALL had occurred during 1956-85 within 3 miles (5 km) of the Winfrith establishment, whereas 2.4 cases would have been expected from the (undeclared) number of cases occurring in the remainder of rural Dorset. No reasons were given either for this choice of radius or for the inclusion of the additional 16 year period before 1972 (the Winfrith site became operational in 1964). The 3 cases were diagnosed between 1977 and 1980, but no prior reason existed for this particular 4 year period of time to be of special interest. Barclay also observed that the highest rates of incidence in the region appeared to occur in commuter communities on the periphery of urban areas, although a preselected analysis structure had not been defined to test for this particular aspect of the geographical distribution of cases.

3.6 Hinkley Point

The Hinkley Point nuclear power station lies on the Somerset coast, and young leukaemia and non-Hodgkin's lymphoma incidence in the area surrounding this station has been the subject of a study by Ewings *et al.* [26]. This study was published at a time when a public inquiry (into the siting of a pressurised water reactor at Hinkley Point) was underway, and in this respect the Ewings *et al.* study is similar to the

1986 Dounreay study of Heasman *et al.* [37]. The "main result" of the study was that the observed number of leukaemia and non-Hodgkin's lymphoma cases occurring during 1964-86 in the population of under 25 year olds living within 12.5 km of Hinkley Point was greater than the number expected from national registration rates (O/E = 19/10.4, p = 0.011). The 12.5 km radius was selected on the basis of the study of Heasman *et al.* [37], and the time period because the station was commissioned in 1964.

Ewings *et al.* investigated the sensitivity of this main result to choice of radius, time period and disease type (leukaemia, NHL, or both). No unusual pattern emerged, apart from the leukaemia and NHL registration ratio for 1969-73 (O/E = 9/2.3, p = 0.0006), although there was no prior reason to single out this particular period of time as being of special interest. Unfortunately, Ewings *et al.* did not follow COMARE's lead [9] and check sensitivity to age group. Taylor [61] has pointed out that the excess during 1964-86 is largely confined to the 15-24 year age group (O/E = 10/3.1, p = 0.001), whereas previous studies had indicated that the 0-14 year age group would have been of most interest. The interpretation of this excess in young adults is unclear, but Taylor suggested that an examination of the exact diagnoses of the cases might be worthwhile.

Earlier reports by Somerset Health Authority researchers (Ewings and Bowie) had identified leukaemia incidence at all ages as being raised throughout Somerset [26], and the study of Ewings *et al.* also shows that the 0-24 year age group leukaemia and NHL registration ratio during 1964-86 for Somerset beyond the 12.5 km radius area around Hinkley Point is raised (O/E = 118/99.9, p<0.05). The ratio for the area associated with Hinkley Point and that for the remainder of Somerset do not differ significantly. Indeed, the ratio for the whole of Somerset during 1959-63 (ie. before the Hinkley Point station was operational) was raised (O/E = 29/17.9, 95% CI = 1.08 to 2.32). The authors remark that [26, p291]:

> "the rates around Hinkley Point may simply have been reflecting high rates throughout Somerset".

Alexander *et al.* [1] have raised a number of points concerning the study of Ewings *et al.* They note that evidence exists for registration data being more complete for the south west region of England than for the country as a whole, and that this effect could contribute to the excess of registered cases near Hinkley Point. They also note that the Hinkley Point study was carried out with the knowledge that leukaemia rates for Somerset were unusually high. Under these circumstances, Alexander *et al.* consider that the most appropriate comparison is the Hinkley Point area with the remainder of Somerset, which does not produce a significant difference of ratios. They conclude [1]:

> "The current results are consistent with a random distribution within Somerset of an excess number of cases, and so undue concern about Hinkley Point should not be aroused".

Since Hinkley Point is just one of a number of similar nuclear power stations in Britain, a study employing data from the area around all such stations would produce more reliable results than a study involving just one site, which may have arisen out of prior knowledge concerning the area. Indeed, one has to ask whether the study would have been carried out had this prior information been absent, or whether the result for Hinkley Point would have been reported in this fashion had it been "negative". The study of Ewings *et al.* is very similar in these respects to the Aldermaston and Burghfield study of Roman *et al.* [50].

3.7 *The Major Installations of England and Wales*

In the early 1980s, Baron, who was working at the Department of Community Medicine and General Practice at Oxford University, undertook a descriptive study of cancer mortality trends in areas around the 15 major nuclear installations in England and Wales [4]. Areas associated with these installations were defined by pre-1974 Local Authority Areas (LAAs) having over half their area lying within 5 miles of the establishment, although there were some exceptions [4]. Where possible, mortality ratios for a number of malignancy types for the 5 year period immediately prior to the commencement of operations at an installation were compared with the equivalent ratios for the 10 or 15 year (depending on data availability) period after this date. In addition, trends of mortality ratios with time after installation "start-up" were examined. (An interesting feature of this study is that similar analyses were performed for 5 non-nuclear power stations situated in non-urban areas of England and Wales:) Baron concluded [4, p823]:

> "In summary, the data described here indicate no generalized trend of rising cancer mortality in small areas around the major facilities in England and Wales".

The Office of Population Censuses and Surveys (OPCS) and the Imperial Cancer Research Fund (ICRF) Cancer Epidemiology and Clinical Trials Unit at Oxford decided to collaborate in an extension of the work by Baron, and the detailed and extensive findings of this study were published in 1987 as an OPCS Report (Cook-Mozaffari *et al.*, [12]). The study used both OPCS cancer mortality and registration data from the 22 year period 1959-1980 for LAAs with at least one-third of their population living within 10 miles of the 15 major nuclear installations in England and Wales, and also for groupings of coastal LAAs to the north and south of Sellafield. In addition, data for matched control LAAs situated away from installations were obtained for the study. The LAA was the smallest unit for which appropriate data were readily available. A wide variety of cancer types, a number of age groups, and distance and temporal data subsets were employed in the various analyses. A more detailed summary of the structure of the OPCS-ICRF study has been given by Forman *et al.* [27], and we have given further details elsewhere [69].

Cook-Mozaffari *et al.* considered that [12, pxi]:
"The main purpose of the statistics generated by this investigation is to provide descriptive material on the patterns of incidence and mortality round nuclear installations."

As such [12, p51]:
"The tests of significance have been used in the present examination of material merely as one way of identifying results for further scrutiny."

There is no doubt that the OPCS Report represents the most detailed and comprehensive study of the available data on cancer incidence and mortality in the vicinity of nuclear establishments carried out to date.

The strengths of the OPCS-ICRF study are:

1) A consistent analysis framework is applied to each nuclear site so that boundaries are not influenced by any previous information on cancer incidence or mortality around particular sites.
2) All major nuclear installations in England and Wales are included so that overall patterns of incidence and mortality may be assessed, and the selective reporting of results for individual installations (perhaps on the basis of prior knowledge) is avoided.
3) Groupings of similar installations (such as the CEGB nuclear power stations) may be constructed. Not only does this avoid the problem of selective reporting, but also the number of multiple comparisons will be reduced, so limiting the number of "false positive" (type I error) results, and the statistical power of each comparison will be increased by employing larger expected numbers. The grouping of installations also overcomes, to some extent, the difficulty of having to use the rather large LAAs as the fundamental geographical units of data acquisition, which

can lead to areas of an unusual shape around some individual installations.

4) The use of both cancer registration and mortality data provides a useful check on the possible presence of data biases (such as variable registration efficiency).
5) The use of data from control areas provides further insight into the possible variation of data quality which might not be revealed through the use of standardised ratios for installation areas alone.

A number of general observations may be made on the results of the OPCS Report.

1) Two major groupings of installations (and their control areas) were identified by Cook-Mozaffari *et al.*: the 5 "pre-1955 installations" that commenced operations before 1955 (Amersham, Harwell, Springfields, Aldermaston and Capenhurst); and the 8 CECB Magnox nuclear power stations (Bradwell, Berkeley and Oldbury, Hinkley, Trawsfynydd, Dungeness, Sizewell and Wylfa). Winfrith was treated separately because it does not fall into either of the two major categories, and Sellafield was also considered on its own because of the scale of the discharges and because of the hypothesis-generating nature of the Sellafield data. It is of interest that, whereas the 8 CEGB power stations form a coherent grouping in terms of function and environmental impact, the pre-1955 installations are a heterogeneous grouping with little in common except age. Because of this, Cook-Mozaffari *et al.* [12] have commented that it would be (p32):

   "surprising if a common effect were found for the pre-1955 installations".

2) Cook-Mozaffari [11] has pointed out that registration ratios for the pre-1955 installation area are consistently greater than the corresponding mortality ratios, but that this phenomenon is not observed in the control area. This and other patterns in the data for this grouping suggested to Cook-Mozaffari that cancer registration data for LAAs in the vicinity of pre-1955 installations are especially complete. Since the pre-1955 installation area accounts for about 80% of the population considered to be living near a nuclear installation, this registration bias will affect the whole dataset [11]. This finding has led those involved in subsequent investigations [27], [13] to use mortality data only, to avoid bias due to variations in registration efficiency.
3) Forman *et al.* [27] have defined a "relative risk (RR)" statistic as being an installation area mortality ratio divided by the corresponding control area mortality ratio. These authors noted that when the overall number of RRs significantly greater than unity is compared with the

overall number of RRs significantly less than unity, there are substantially less "positive" results than there are "negative" results. Although Forman *et al.* found this finding reassuring in terms of the general level of cancer risk in the vicinity of nuclear installations, they pointed out that this also indicates that appreciable differences in the background levels of cancer risk factors exist between installation and control areas, making the interpretation of any particular RR problematical.

Cook-Mozaffari *et al.* concluded that [12, p87]:

"Consideration of apparent biases in registration between installation locations compared with control, of the patterns of results for mortality rather than incidence, and of the results for control locations strongly suggests that the positive results for nuclear installations are predomonantly due to data biases and to random fluctuations rather than local environment".

Given that the Black Group found evidence of raised leukaemia incidence and mortality rates for young people living near Sellafield [40], of particular interest amongst the results of the OPCS-ICRF study must be the young leukaemia mortality RRs for those installation groupings which do not include Sellafield. (In fact, the OPCS Report gives a 0-24 year old leukaemia mortality RR for Sellafield of 0.88 (95% CI 0.46-1.71), which reflects the longer time period and larger geographical area considered in this study when compared with the young leukaemia mortality studies provided to the Black Group [40] - see Subsection 3.1). The 0-24 year old leukaemia mortality installation O/Es and RRs are [30]:

Grouping	Installation O/E	95% CI	RR	95% CI
Sellafield	1.26	0.76-1.95	0.88	0.46-1.71
pre-1955	0.99	0.89-1.09	0.94	0.82-1.07
CEGB	1.11	0.88-1.34	1.13	0.83-1.55
Winfrith	1.13	0.71-1.71	0.90	0.49-1.67
All except Sellafield	1.02	0.93-1.11	0.96	0.85-1.08

So, the statistics of most interest do not reveal any unusual result, although the relatively large area associated with the installations must be borne in mind. The results of an examination of trends of RR with distance zone and time period were also unremarkable [12], [27].

However, Forman *et al.* [27] have noted that if data for lymphoid leukaemia mortality in the 0-24 year age group are extracted from the OPCS Report, then some noteworthy results are obtained. (Lymphoid leukaemia deaths could be separated out from all leukaemia deaths only for the period 1968-1980). We have discussed these results in more detail elsewhere [69], but the finding of most interest is the young lymphoid leukaemia mortality RR for the innermost distance zone of the pre-1955 installation grouping: RR=2.10, $p<0.01$.

One of the difficulties of interpreting this result is that the raised RR is predominantly due to an exceptionally low mortality ratio in the control area (installation O/E = 42/37.0; control O/E = 20/37.0). Given that differences exist between installation and control areas that can affect overall levels of cancer mortality, this particular RR must be treated with caution, especially because of the diverse nature of the pre-1955 installations [69]. In addition, it might be considered that the primary results of interest as far as hypothesis-testing is concerned are for all leukaemia mortality in the 0-24 year age group during 1959-80, and these results are not unusual. The lymphoid leukaemia findings are a subset of these results, albeit findings which require further study. It must also be noted that Forman *et al.* were obliged to employ mortality rather than incidence data, which could lead to some distortion of results for the period 1968-80, when childhood ALL was being treated with increasing success.

Recently, Cook-Mozaffari *et al.* [13] have adopted an alternative approach to the use of control areas, in an effort to avoid RRs which reflect differences in the levels of background risk factors in installation and control areas. In this latest study, cancer mortality data for the 402 post-1974 County Districts (CDs) of England and Wales for the 10 year period 1969-1978 were employed. This structure was essentially dictated by the nature of the available data [13]. A log-linear regression analysis has been carried out to determine RRs for areas around nuclear installations whilst accounting for variation due to four background factors: social class, rural status, population size and health authority region. (It will be noted that these four variables apply to districts rather than to individuals, and that they therefore act as surrogates for correlated variations in levels of individual risk factors). In this study, a district was considered to be associated with an installation if at least 0.1% of its population lies within a 10 mile radius, although three distance zones were also considered.

The regression analysis was successful in removing most of the anomalous RRs noted by Forman *et al.* [27], and which were presumably due to matching deficiencies; but the adjustment process had little impact upon the 0-24 year old leukaemia mortality RRs [30]:

	Unadjusted		Adjusted	
Grouping	RR	95% CI	RR	95% CI
Sellafield	1.72	0.93-3.18	1.85	0.98-3.49
pre-1955	1.14	1.04-1.26	1.14	1.00-1.31
CEGB	1.08	0.92-1.25	1.15	0.97-1.36
Winfrith	0.87	0.54-1.39	0.96	0.58-1.58
All except Sellafield	1.11	1.02-1.21	1.14	1.02-1.26

The differences between these results and those of the OPCS Report (tabulated earlier in this subsection) are due to:

1) The OPCS Report [12] uses the period 1959-80, whereas the later Cook-Mozaffari *et al.* study [13] uses 1969-78.
2) The OPCS Report uses pre-1974 LAAs, whereas the later study uses districts based upon post-1974 CDs, which leads to different areas being associated with installations.
3) The OPCS Report uses control areas to account for variations in background factors, whereas the later study adjusts expected numbers using regression analysis of mortality rates throughout England and Wales.

Most of the excess leukaemia deaths are due to lymphoid leukaemia, so it would appear that the findings of Forman *et al.* [27] are not just a peculiarity of the control area mortality ratios.

Whilst the latest study of Cook-Mozaffari *et al.* [13] provides evidence of a generally elevated level of young leukaemia mortality in areas associated with nuclear installations, it should be noted that the post-1974 CDs, upon which the study is based, are generally larger than pre-1974 LAAs. This means that the areas associated with installations in this study are quite sizeable geographical units, that extend (sometimes considerably) beyond 10 miles from an establishment [13, p477, Figure 1]. It is difficult to envisage how site operations can directly influence the risk of young leukaemia over such relatively large areas in any meaningful way, particularly since the trend analysis carried out in the study shows that the RR for a district appears not to be related to the size of population living within 10 miles of an installation. However, alternative explanations are not obvious.

One further noteworthy finding of the recent Cook-Mozaffari *et al.* study is that the regression analysis of young leukaemia mortality rates for all the districts of England and Wales revealed a significant ($p<0.01$) positive trend of RR with increasing proportion of the population of a district being of higher socioeconomic class. This trend is due to the distribution of the lymphoid leukaemia RR rather than the other leukaemias RR. Lymphoid leukaemia mortality also displayed a significant ($p<0.05$) variation with health authority region.

It is of note that even after account had been taken of variations in young leukaemia RR due to the four factors incorporated in the regression analysis, the degree of remaining variation was still significantly greater than would be expected from an adjusted Poisson distribution of deaths between districts. This (unquantified) extra-Poisson variation is presumably due to the geographical non-uniformity of risk factors other than those dealt with through the use of the four socioeconomic and demographic variables. The extra-Poisson variation was greatest for young lymphoid leukaemia mortality. We shall return to the important subject of the underlying (background) distribution of leukaemia cases in the final section.

3.8 Nuclear Installations Outside Britain

A number of small-scale studies of cancer incidence/mortality around nuclear establishments in the USA have been reported [63], [30], but few of these have dealt with childhood leukaemia. The results of a large study of cancer mortality in the vicinity of the major nuclear installations of the USA, which is currently being carried out by researchers from the National Cancer Institute, should be available in 1990.

The study of cancer mortality around the La Hague nuclear facilities on the Normandy coast of France illustrates the problems of interpretation associated with the analysis of data from sparsely populated areas. During 1970-82, no deaths from leukaemia amongst the 0-24 year old age group occurred in the Beaumont-Hague canton (containing the La Hague establishment), whereas 0.72 deaths would have been expected from the leukaemia mortality experience of the Manche department as a whole [23]. (This expected number is based upon 48 deaths). However, the upper 95% confidence limit for

O/E which may be derived from these data is 5, so that the observation of zero deaths is compatible with up to a fivefold relative risk in this canton. Unfortunately, it could be difficult to improve upon this precision without the inclusion of communities which may be irrelevant to the possible increased risk under consideration.

3.9 The Rural New Towns of Britain

Kinlen [44] noted that the Sellafield and Dounreay establishments were located in isolated areas that had experienced a large influx of population as a result of the employment demands of the sites. He suggested that if childhood leukaemia is a rare response to a common infective agent, then the unusual patterns of infection generated by large numbers of people moving into isolated communities could cause an increase in the risk of childhood leukaemia in these areas. Kinlen initially tested this hypothesis using data from the Kirkcaldy District of Fife, which contains Glenrothes New Town. During the 1950s Glenrothes grew rapidly, and the district was moderately secluded before the opening of the Forth Road Bridge in 1964. The Glenrothes area during the 1950s and early 1960s was considered by Kinlen to be the only area of Scotland sufficiently similar to Thurso (near Dounreay) in terms of isolation and population influx for a test of hypothesis to be carried out.

Leukaemia and lymphoma mortality data for the 0-24 year old age group were collected for Kirkcaldy District for the years 1951 to 1985, with the first half of the time period (1951-67) being of primary interest. During 1951-67, the observed number of young leukaemia deaths was significantly in excess of the expected number ($O/E = 10/3.6$, $p<0.01$). If non-Hodgkin's lymphoma deaths were added to the leukaemia deaths, the excess remained highly significant ($O/E = 11/4.4$, $p<0.01$). Most of the excess of young leukaemia and NHL deaths occurred in the 0-4 year age group (O=8, E=1.8), and Kinlen observed that the majority of these deaths occurred in the period before 1960. During 1968-85, there was no excess of leukaemia and NHL deaths in Kirkcaldy District (O=2, E=6.3).

It is of interest that Kinlen also gathered data for Thurso, and that during 1951-67 no significant excess of young leukaemia and NHL deaths occurred (O=2, E=1.5). It might have been anticipated that Thurso would also have experienced an enhanced risk in this earlier period, the data for which had not previously been examined. However, the expected number of deaths in the Glenrothes area during 1951-67 is 4.4, compared with 1.5 for Thurso, giving a 95% confidence interval for the mortality ratio for Glenrothes as 1.3-4.5, and for

Thurso as 0.2-4.8. The 1951-67 mortality ratio for Thurso is not incompatible with that for the Glenrothes area.

The important difference between the Glenrothes study and some of the other studies reviewed in this paper is that it had not been prompted by previous suspicions of an excess of childhood leukaemia cases in the area, and that boundaries had been selected in the absence of prior knowledge of the data. Kinlen has noted [44, p1326]:

> "The Glenrothes cluster of childhood leukaemia seems to be the first instance of a particular cluster being found as predicted by a hypothesis specified before the data were collected".

Kinlen [45] has also presented preliminary findings from a study of four new towns constructed during the late 1940s and the early 1950s in largely rural areas of England and Wales: Aycliffe, Corby, Cwmbran and Peterlee. Since the Glenrothes excess was mainly due to deaths in young children before 1960, Kinlen examined the 0-4 year old leukaemia mortality data for this group of four towns for the period from the start of the growth of each new town up to 1960. A significant excess of leukaemia deaths was found: O/E = 10/3.1, $p<0.01$. Kinlen has concluded [45, p277]:

> "Evidence is therefore mounting that childhood leukaemia originates in some type of infective process and that certain types of population mixing are conducive to its occurrence. Strong reasons would be required for supposing that this effect did not operate near nuclear reprocessing sites, so unusual is their demographic pattern".

Kinlen's studies are excellent examples of hypothesis-testing carried out with no interference of prior knowledge upon the study design. They also illustrate the difficulties of studying childhood leukaemia incidence near nuclear installations when major causal factors (and therefore major confounding factors) remain unknown.

4. CONCLUDING REMARKS

It is clear that the Seascale childhood leukaemia (plus, perhaps, non-Hodgkin's lymphoma) incidence rate has been unusually high over at least the last three decades; but the excess of cases seems to have been largely confined to this village in the vicinity of Sellafield. The nature of the discovery of the Seascale "cluster" has led to much debate over its interpretation, with no satisfactory conclusion as yet. However, the Seascale observation has generated a (rather broad) hypothesis for testing using independent data, and this has been done, although not without difficulty, in a number of studies. Despite problems in the manner in which the analysis of data from the Dounreay area has been conducted, it does appear as though a significant excess of childhood leukaemia cases has occurred around this establishment. The evidence from studies of other individual areas is less convincing, primarily because of the influence of prior knowledge of data. However, the study of areas around all the major nuclear installations of England and Wales, carried out, most recently, by Cook-Mozaffari *et al.* [13], does indicate that young leukaemia mortality has been generally higher than expected around nuclear sites. Again, interpretation is not straightforward because of the large areas apparently affected, and the lack of trend of mortality rate with distance from an installation. The explanation for the observed patterns of childhood leukaemia incidence and mortality is liable to be a complex one - for example, Kinlen [44], [45] has suggested that the case excesses at Seascale and around Dounreay may be due, at least in part, to the unusual population mixing caused by the presence of large establishments in remote and sparsely populated areas, and he has shown that childhood leukaemia mortality was higher than expected in those rural new towns where population mixing in the 1950s was particularly extreme.

If the major factors in the aetiology of the childhood leukaemias are not distributed uniformly in space and time, then deviations from an underlying age-sex adjusted Poisson process may be capable of being detected. The nature of such deviations, if present, may provide clues as to the identity of important background risk factors, and the levels of these factors around nuclear installations will be relevant to the rates of incidence in these areas. In the 1960s and 1970s, a considerable interest developed in whether space-time clustering of childhood leukaemia cases occurs, primarily motivated by speculation that childhood leukaemia might be weakly infective. The studies

> "failed to produce convincing evidence of clustering of the leukemias" [53, p406],

but the methods employed may not have been sufficiently sensitive to detect particular forms of clustering [7]. More recently, a number of studies have looked for departures of the observed geographical distribution of young leukaemia cases or deaths, from that expected from a Poisson process. At the time of the Black Inquiry, Gardner and Winter examined the distribution of 0-24 year old leukaemia deaths between 152 similarly-sized Rural Districts of England and Wales during 1968-78, and they failed to find a significant deviation from a Poisson distribution [40], [30]. Heasman *et al.* carried out a similar analysis of the distribution of 0-24 year old leukaemia registrations between the 898 postcode sectors of Scotland during 1968-84, and found a distribution consistent with that expected from a Poisson process [38]. Wakeford also examined these data, and did not detect a significantly larger than expected number of high rates of incidence [67]. Following a suggestion by Wilkie at a public inquiry [73], Scottish Health Service researchers have re-examined these registration data using areas of approximately equal expected numbers of cases, but this analysis failed to change the original "negative" findings [9].

These analyses are largely based upon the comparison of observed and expected distributions using a chi-squared test. Cook-Mozaffari *et al.* [13] have adopted a different approach, and have examined the distribution of 0-24 year old leukaemia deaths between 400 districts of England and Wales during 1969-78 using a regression analysis. They found significant extra-Poisson variability (see Subsection 3.7). The apparent contradiction between these recent findings and those of earlier studies may be due to differences in statistical power, and the power of the methods has yet to be studied in detail. A lot of work on the background distribution of childhood leukaemia cases is currently underway [52], and it will be of interest to see the results. Of equal importance is the development of a high quality childhood cancer incidence national database [10], which will avoid the problems of using presently available registration data and of using mortality data.

It is of note that the epidemiological studies of childhood leukaemia incidence and/or mortality around nuclear installations carried out so far have been "ecological studies" - the study group has been defined by geographical proximity to an establishment, but factors relating to individuals have not been investigated. The case-control studies presently in progress will rectify this situation; but it will be important to maintain the distinction between hypothesis generation and testing in these studies.

Hopefully the effort being expended on the study of childhood leukaemia will soon yield results, and lead to a clarification of the statistical association between childhood leukaemia incidence and nuclear establishments. If these investigations have quickened the pace of advancement of the basic understanding of the childhood leukaemias, with the benefits to medical practice that this should bring, then the effort will have been worthwhile.

REFERENCES

[1] Alexander, F.E., Cartwright, R.A., McKinney, P.A. and Ricketts, T.J., (1989) Incidence of Leukaemia in Vicinity of Hinkley Point Nuclear Power Station, *British Medical Journal*, **229**, 565.

[2] Barclay, R., (1986) Childhood Leukaemia in West Berkshire, *Lancet*, **i**, 212.

[3] Barclay, R., (1987) Childhood Leukaemia in Wessex, *Community Medicine*, **9**, 279-285.

[4] Baron, J.A., (1984) Cancer Mortality in Small Areas around Nuclear Facilities in England and Wales, *British Journal of Cancer*, **50**, 815-824.

[5] Barton, C.J., Roman, E., Ryder, H.M. and Watson, A., (1985) Childhood Leukaemia in West Berkshire, *Lancet*, **ii**, 1248-1249.

[6] Bithell, J.F. and Stone, R.A., (1989) On Statistical Methods of Analysing the Geographical Distribution of Cancer Cases near Nuclear Installations, *Journal of Epidemiology and Community Health*, **43**, 79-85.

[7] Chen, R., Mantel, N. and Klingberg, M.A., (1984) A Study of Three Techniques for Time-Space Clustering in Hodgkin's Disease, *Statistics in Medicine*, **3**, 173-184.

[8] Committee on Medical Aspects of Radiation in the Environment (COMARE), "First Report", Her Majesty's Stationery Office, London, 1986.

[9] Committee on Medical Aspects of Radiation in the Environment (COMARE), "Second Report", Her Majesty's Stationery Office, London, 1988.

[10] Committee on Medical Aspects of Radiation in the Environment (COMARE), "Third Report", Her Majesty's Stationery Office, London, 1989.

[11] Cook-Mozaffari, P., (1987) Cancer Near Nuclear Installations, *Lancet*, **i**, 855-856.

[12] Cook-Mozaffari, P.J., Ashwood, F.L., Vincent, T., Forman, D. and Alderson, M., (1987) "Cancer Incidence and Mortality in the Vicinity of Nuclear Installations, England and Wales, 1959-80," Studies on Medical and Population Subjects No. 51, Her Majesty's Stationery Office, London.

[13] Cook-Mozaffari, P.J., Darby, S.C., Doll, R., Forman, D., Hermon, C., Pike, M.C. and Vincent, T., (1989) Geographical Variation in Mortality from Leukaemia and Other Cancers in England and Wales in Relation to Proximity to Nuclear Installations, 1969-78, *British Journal of Cancer,* **59**, 476-485.

[14] Craft, A.W., Openshaw, S. and Birch, J.M., (1984) Apparent Clusters of Childhood Lymphoid Malignancy in Northern England, *Lancet,* **i** , 96-97.

[15] Craft, A.W. Openshaw, S. and Birch J.M., (1985) Childhood Cancer in the Northern Region, 1968-82: Incidence in Small Geographical Areas, *Journal of Epidemiology and Community Health,* **39**, 53-57.

[16] Croasdale, M.R. and White, A.A.L., (1988) A Critical Review of Statistical Evaluations of the Clustering of Rare Diseases with Particular Application to the Frequency of Clusters around Nuclear Sites in Great Britain, In "Health Effects of Low Dose Ionising Radiation - Recent Advances and their Implications," pp145-149, British Nuclear Energy Society, London.

[17] Cutler, J., (1983) British Nuclear Foul-up Limited, *New Statesman,* 18 November, pp8-10.

[18] Cuzick, J., (1985) Searching for Clusters and Associations in Cancer Epidemiology, *Leukemia Research,* **9**, 669-670.

[19] Davies, J.M. and Inskip, H., (1986) "Epidemiological Studies of General Population Groups Exposed to Low-Level Radiation," Organisation for Economic Cooperation and Development, Paris.

[20] Dionian, J., Muirhead, C.R., Wan, S.L. and Wrixon, A.D., (1986) "The Risks of Leukaemia and Other Cancers in Thurso from Radiation Exposure," Report NRPB-R196, Her Majesty's Stationary Office, London.

[21] Dionian, J., Wan, S.L. and Wrixon, A.D., (1987) "Radiation Doses to Members of the Public around AWRE Aldermaston, ROF Burghfield and AERE Harwell", Report NRPB-R202, Her Majesty's Stationery Office, London.

[22] Doll, R., (1989) The Epidemiology of Childhood Leukaemia *Journal of the Royal Statistical Society,* Series A, **152**, 341-351.

[23] Dousset, M., (1989) Cancer Mortality around La Hague Nuclear Facilities, *Health Physics*, **56**, 875-884.

[24] Ennis, J.R., (1987) How Should the Health of Communities near Nuclear Installations be Monitored? *Journal of the Society of Occupational Medicine*, **37**, 19-23.

[25] Enterline, P.E., (1985) Evaluating Cancer Clusters, *American Industrial Hygiene Association Journal*, **46**, B10-B13.

[26] Ewings, P.D., Bowie, C., Phillips, M.J. and Johnson, S.A.N., (1989) Incidence of Leukaemia in Young People in the Vicinity of Hinkley Point Nuclear Power Station, 1959-86, *British Medical Journal*, **299**, 289-293.

[27] Forman, D., Cook-Mozaffari, P., Darby, S., Davey, G., Stratton, I., Doll, R. and Pike, M., (1987) Cancer near Nuclear Installations, *Nature*, **329**, 499-505.

[28] Gallop, R.G.C., Warren, B.B., Hannan, A.M. and Saxby, W.N., (1988) The Control of the Exposure of the General Public to Radioactive Materials in the Environs of the Atomic Weapons Research Establishment (AWRE) Aldermaston, In "Health Effects of Low Dose Ionising Radiation - Recent Advances and their Implications", pp189-191, and pp 206-207, British Nuclear Energy Society, London.

[29] Gardner, M.J., (1985) Childhood Cancer in West Cumbria, *Lancet*, **i**, 403-404.

[30] Gardner, M.J., (1989) Review of Reported Increases of Childhood Cancer Rates in the Vicinity of Nuclear Installations in the UK, *Journal of the Royal Statistical Society*, Series A, **152**, 307-325.

[31] Gardner, M.J., Hall, A.J., Downes, S. and Terrell, J.D., (1987) Follow up Study of Children Born Elsewhere but Attending Schools in Seascale, West Cumbria (Schools Cohort), *British Medical Journal*, **295**, 819-822.

[32] Gardner, M.J., Hall, A.J., Downes, S. and Terrell, J.D., (1987) Follow up Study of Children Born to Mothers Resident in Seascale, West Cumbria (Birth Cohort), *British Medical Journal*, **295**, 822-827.

[33] Gardner, M.J. and Winter, P.D., (1984) Mortality in Cumberland during 1959-78 with Reference to Cancer in Young People around Windscale, *Lancet*, **i**, 216-217.

[34] Glass, A.G., Hill, J.A. and Miller, R.W., (1968) Significance of Leukemia Clusters, *Journal of Pediatrics*, **73**, 101-107.

[35] Hargreaves, R., Wilkie, D. and Wakeford, R., (1988) A Re-Examination of the Epidemiological Data for Cumbrian Coastal Areas, In "Health Effects of Low Dose Ionising Radiation - Recent Advances and their Implications," pp125-131, British Nuclear Energy Society, London.

[36] Heasman, M.A., Kemp, I.W., MacLaren, A.M., Trotter, P., Gillis, C.R. and Hole, D.J., (1984) Incidence of Leukaemia in Young Persons in West of Scotland, *Lancet*, **i**, 1188-1189, 1310.

[37] Heasman, M.A., Kemp, I.W., Urquhart, J.D. and Black, R., (1986) Childhood Leukaemia in Northern Scotland, *Lancet*, **i**, 266, 385.

[38] Heasman, M.A., Urquhart, J.D., Black, R.J., Kemp, I.W., Glass, S. and Gray, M., (1987) Leukaemia in Young Persons in Scotland: a Study of its Geographical Distribution and Relationship to Nuclear Installations, *Health Bulletin*, **45**, 147-151.

[39] Hutchison D., (1985) Statistical Significance Testing and the Black Report on Sellafield, *Radical Statistics Newsletter*, **34**, 1-18.

[40] Independent Advisory Group (Chairman: Sir Douglas Black), Investigation of the Possible Increased Incidence of Cancer in West Cumbria, Her Majesty's Stationery Office, London, (1984).

[41] Independent Committee (Chairman: Professor W.S.B. Lowry), Investigation into Patterns of Disease with Possible Association with Radiation in Northern Ireland, Her Majesty's Stationery Office, Belfast, (1989).

[42] Jessop, E.G. and Horsley, S.D., (1985) Multiple Myeloma in South Cumbria 1974-80: Problems of Health Analysis in Small Communities, *Journal of Epidemiology and Community Health*, **39**, 231-236.

[43] Jones, D.R. and Rushton, L., (1982) Simultaneous Inference in Epidemiological Studies, *International Journal of Epidemiology*, **11**, 276-282.

[44] Kinlen, L., (1988) Evidence for an Infective Cause of Childhood Leukaemia: Comparison of a Scottish New Town with Nuclear Reprocessing Sites in Britain, *Lancet*, **ii**, 1323-1326.

[45] Kinlen, L., (1989) The Relevance of Population Mixing to the Aetiology of Childhood Leukaemia, In " Medical Response to Effects of Ionising Radiation" (eds. W.A. Crosbie and J.H. Gittus), pp272-278, Elsevier, London.

[46] Kyle, R.A., Herber, L., Evatt, B.L. and Heath, C.W., (1970) Multiple Myeloma, a Community Cluster, *Journal of the American Medical Association,* **213**, 1339-1341.

[47] Linet, M.S., (1985) The Leukemias: Epidemiologic Aspects, Oxford University Press, New York.

[48] McPhedran, P. and Heath, C.W., (1969) Multiple Cases of Leukemia Associated with One House, *Journal of the American Medical Association,* **209**, 2021-2025.

[49] Office of Population Censuses and Surveys, " Area Mortality, Decennial Supplement for England and Wales, 1969-73," Series DS No. 4, Her Majesty's Stationery Office, London, (1981).

[50] Roman, E., Beral, V., Carpenter, L., Watson, A., Barton, C., Ryder, H. and Aston, D.L., (1987) Childhood Leukaemia in the West Berkshire and Basingstoke and North Hampshire District Health Authorities in Relation to Nuclear Establishments in the Vicinity, *British Medical Journal,* **294**, 597-602.

[51] Rose, G. and Barker, D.J.P., (1986) "Epidemiology for the Uninitiated," British Medical Journal, London.

[52] Royal Statistical Society Meeting on Cancer near Nuclear Installations, *Journal of the Royal Statistical Society,* Series A, **152**, 305-384, (1989).

[53] Smith, P.G., (1982) Spatial and Temporal Clustering, In "Cancer Epidemiology and Prevention" (eds. D. Schottenfeld and J.F. Fraumeni) pp391-407, Saunders, Philadelphia.

[54] Smith, P.G. and Pike, M.C., (1976) Current Epidemiological Evidence for Transmission of Hodgkin's Disease, *Cancer Research*, **36**, 660-662.

[55] Stather, J.W., Clarke, R.H. and Duncan, K.P., (1988) "The Risk of Childhood Leukaemia near Nuclear Establishments," Report NRPB-R215, Her Majesty's Stationery Office, London.

[56] Stather, J.W., Dionian, J., Brown, J., Fell, T.P. and Muirhead, C.R., (1986) The Risks of Leukaemia and Other Cancers in Seascale from Radiation Exposure, Report NRPB-R171 Addendum, Her Majesty's Stationery Office, London.

[57] Stather, J.W., Dionian, J., Brown, J., Fell, T.P. and Muirhead, C.R., (1988) The Risk of Leukemia in Seascale from Radiation Exposure, *Health Physics*, **55**, 471-481.

[58] Stather, J.W., Wrixon, A.D. and Simmonds, J.R., (1984) "The Risks of Leukaemia and other Cancers in Seascale from Radiation Exposure," Report NRPB-R171, Her Majesty's Stationery Office, London.

[59] Stiller, C.A., (1985) Descriptive Epidemiology of Childhood Leukaemia and Lymphoma in Great Britain, *Leukemia Research*, **9**, 671-674.

[60] Swerdlow, A.J., (1986) Cancer Registration in England and Wales: Some Aspects Relevant to Interpretation of the Data, *Journal of the Royal Statistical Society*, Series A, **149**, 146-160.

[61] Taylor, R.H., (1989) Incidence of Leukaemia in Vicinity of Hinkley Point Nuclear Power Station, *British Medical Journal*, **299**, 565-566.

[62] Thomas, D.C., (1985) The Problem of Multiple Inference in Identifying Point-Source Environmental Hazards, *Environmental Health Perspectives*, **62**, 407-414.

[63] Tokuhata, G.K. and Smith, M.W., (1981) History of Health Studies around Nuclear Facilities: A Methodological Consideration, *Environmental Research*, **25**, 75-86.

[64] Urquhart, J. and Cutler, J.A., (1985) Incidence of Childhood Cancer in West Cumbria, *Lancet*, **i**, 172.

[65] Urquhart, J., Cutler, J., and Burke, M., (1986) Leukaemia and Lymphatic Cancer in Young People near Nuclear Installations, *Lancet*, **i**, 304.

[66] Urquhart, J., Palmer, M. and Cutler, J., (1984) Cancer in Cumbria: the Windscale Connection, *Lancet*, **i**, 217-218.

[67] Wakeford, R., (1987) Letter to the Editor, *Radiological Protection Bulletin*, **83**, 23-24.

[68] Wakeford, R., (1988) Childhood Leukaemia Incidence around Nuclear Installations, *Lancet*, **i**, 309.

[69] Wakeford, R., Binks, K. and Wilkie, D., (1989) Childhood Leukaemia and Nuclear Installations, *Journal of the Royal Statistical Society*, Series A, **152**, 61-86.

[70] Wakeford, R., Dhodakia, R., Binks, K. and Wilkie, D., (1989) Leukaemia "Clusters" and Nuclear Installations with Special Reference to Dounreay, In "Radiation Protection - Theory and Practice "(ed. E.P. Goldfinch), pp75-78, IOP Publishing, Bristol.

[71] Wan, S.L. and Wrixon, A.D., (1988) "Radiation Doses from Coal-Fired Plants in Oxfordshire and Berkshire," Report NRPB-R203, Her Majesty's Stationery Office, London.

[72] Wheldon, T.E., (1989) The Assessment of Risk of Radiation-induced Childhood Leukaemia in the Vicinity of Nuclear Installations, *Journal of the Royal Statistical Society,* Series A, **152**, 327-339.

[73] Wilkie, D., (1986) "Transcripts of Proceedings of the EDRP Inquiry, Thurso, Day 72," pp49, 50, Scottish Office, Edinburgh.

[74] Wrixon, A.D., (1987) Radiation Doses and Risks of Leukaemia around Nuclear Sites, *Radiological Protection Bulletin,* **83**, 6-12.

A NEW APPROACH TO THE DETECTION AND VALIDATION OF CANCER CLUSTERS: A REVIEW OF OPPORTUNITIES, PROGRESS AND PROBLEMS

S. Openshaw
*(Centre for Urban and Regional Development Studies
University of Newcastle)*

1. INTRODUCTION

This paper outlines the development of a computer automated geographical analysis machine (GAM) which has been produced by a geographer as a response to the practical problem of searching a cancer data base for evidence of spatial clustering. It was developed to meet a specific operational need to try and exploit the new opportunities for analysis being created by the appearance of greatly improved health data bases. Attention here is focussed in particular on acute lymphoblastic leukaemia in children, a form of cancer which is of contemporary interest because of a suspected link with low level radiation discharges from nuclear installations, and its key political and highly media-visible role in the continuing debate about nuclear safety in the UK. However, the technology is also of more general utility. It is a data base trawling device that can be used to search for the unexpected. This proactive characteristic is a very important feature for any cancer analysis system.

The need for new, more automated, forms of geographic analysis is a result of vast changes in the amount and spatial detail of health data sets, particularly, cancer registration systems. It is interesting that within the space of a decade, the geographical resolution of these data has changed from Local Authority sized building blocks, to wards, and then to unit postcodes. By the early 1990s it will probably be down to the individual household level. It brings with it a requirement to move from coarse to fine grained cancer atlases, a shift from zonal to point referenced data, and ultimately a desire to predict cancer incidence at the individual level.

This improved geographical resolution reflects the widespread utilisation of postcodes as a means of referencing address data. Postcodes can be converted to ward and local authority areas (using the Central Postcode Directory), to point grid-references with a resolution of 100 metres (via POSTZON), and soon down to 1 metre (via the Postal Address Code), and also via various proprietory systems linkages with a small area census statistics for enumeration districts.

The result is a data rich environment within which various geographical and statistical analyses can be performed. It is important to emphasise, however, that these developments in data provision and geographic resolution have not been matched, or indeed driven by, the development of any more relevant theories of disease causation. It is almost as if there is now a requirement to analyse the data purely because it exists. Indeed, many of the people involved (viz clinicians) have no clear idea of what types of analyses they want from their data, other than a check on some vaguely defined notions that some unusual spatial or space-time patterns may exists. It is important to also emphasise that the nature of the data tends to limit the type of analysis that can be applied to some kind of geographic epidemiological style of investigation. The data bases whilst rich in a geographical sense also tend to be deficient and quite limited in terms of the available range of variables likely to be of interest in a search for improved, casual understanding.

The aim then is to explore data in search of evidence of spatial pattern. This approach can be readily justified on the grounds that the natural history of many diseases, particularly leukaemia, is so little understood that it is very difficult to specify either many or any sensible a prior hypotheses. Moreover, as the paper by Wakefield, Binks and Wilkie (see this volume) demonstrates, there are a number of critical operational difficulties that confront more traditional hypothesis-testing studies and undermine their scientific validity in this context.

Section 2 briefly describes the design of a mark I prototype geographical analysis machine and reviews its use as a means of searching for evidence of spatial clustering using child cancer registration data for Northern England. In Section 3 an attempt is made to validate the results that were obtained. Finally, Section 4 outlines the development of other GAM variants as a response to an improved understanding of the operational characteristics of the classic GAM/1 procedure.

2. AUTOMATING THE SEARCH FOR CANCER CLUSTERS

2.1 The design of a prototype GAM

The basic idea that resulted in the development of the first GAM is very simple and was a direct result of reading Wilkie's evidence at the 1986-7 Dounreay Fast Reactor Reprocessing Plant Public Inquiry (Wilkie, 1986). The complaint was made that the evidence presented at the Inquiry by the Information Services Division of the Scottish Health Service Common Service Agency (see Wakefield, Binks, and Wilkie - this volume) was biased by an unfortunate albeit unintentional combination of boundary gerrymandering and post-hoc hypothesis testing. It is noted that in that study population and cancer data was obtained for a circular study region and a Poisson probability used to assess whether the observed number of cancers could have occurred by chance. With this technique there are a number of key operational decisions which have a major impact on the results:

(1) The selection of a point source to be investigated on the basis of a prior hypothesis;

(2) The prior selection of a particular radius for the circular study region for which a measure of significance is to be obtained;

(3) The prior selection of a specific time period for the study; and

(4) The prior selection of either a particular disease or grouping of diseases.

One solution to these problems is to use a properly specified, predetermined, analysis structure and within this framework try to devise significance tests of greater power. The alternative is to automate the entire process and then to systematically explore the universe of results that can be obtained by identifying and examining all combinations of these four key operational decisions. Instead of only examining one or two locations thought to be of particular a priori interest, why not examine all locations. Instead of specifying a specific radius, why not examine a wide spectrum of alternative radii; instead of selecting a particular time subgrouping why not examine all alternatives; and do likewise for the various disease categorisations considered relevant. This universe of potential results will contain all knowledge both known and unknown relating to the data and the generic hypothesis being evaluated; it is locationally unbiased in that all locations are treated equally; it is independent of any zoning system, and prior knowledge of the data is no longer considered relevant since such knowledge is not used.

However, there are a number of problems in adopting this style of analysis. Particular mention is made of the need to evaluate perhaps several millions (and even tens of millions) of hypotheses, the need to take into account the locational and representational uncertainties contained in the geographic data being analysed, the complexity of multiple perhaps non-independent significance testing and lack of knowledge of their properties, and the dependency of the results on the (unknown) power of whatever test statistic is used. The first problem is overcome either by extended run times or by coding the procedure for a supercomputer. The second problem is handled by a form of auto-sensitivity analysis. The other problems were ignored because the initially limited objective was to develop what was considered to be a purely geographical pattern descriptive technique which puts less emphasis on these latter aspects than a more statistical approach would have required. It was also thought that they could be explored via simulation at a later date. At the same time this new approach was little more than an extrapolation of traditional practice where such detailed statistical questions were not usually investigated and this study differed mainly in the geographical detail that was introduced. The aim was to merely identify potentially anomalous locations to be investigated further by a different style of analysis.

2.2 Building a GAM/1

The basic idea of taking a particular generic hypothesis (viz the probability that the observed number of cancers within a circle of radius (r) at point (x,y) could have occurred by chance) and then building an analysis machine by generalising the spatial and locational components can be operationalised in a number of ways. In the route selected for GAM/1 there are four key components:

(1) a means of generating the universe of hypotheses of a particular generic type;

(2) a means of detecting pattern involving a test statistic and a significance assessment procedure;

(3) a means of reporting the results; and

(4) a Geographic Information System (GIS) to handle all the spatial data retrieval requests.

A full description of these aspects is provided in Openshaw et al. (1987) and only scant details are given here.

The one key operational decision that needs to be made concerns the nature of the generic hypothesis. GAM/1 uses a circular region of interest (reflecting its historic origins) and is concerned with identifying the subset of all circles that have a sufficiently excess cancer count to be significantly different from what would have been expected had the cancer of interest been randomly distributed throughout the population at risk in the study region. This assessment was initially made using a Monte Carlo significance test. The test statistic was a cancer count and this was assessed using 499 different, population at risk weighted, random cancer distributions. A Monte Carlo significance test was used to provide for subsequent flexibility in changing the nature of the null hypothesis; viz to consider various forms of random clustering or variation in registration efficiency, and to allow different test statistics to be used. However, virtually identical results are obtained if an analytical Poisson calculation is used instead of simulation.

The locational component of this generic hypothesis is varied in a systematic manner by covering the study region with a lattice. Circles of a given radius are generated about each lattice intersection. The lattice is spaced sufficiently close relative to the radius of the circles being examined, so that the circles overlap by a large degree. A lattice spacing of circle radii was considered appropriate. It is important that the circles overlap in order to provide a good discrete approximation to considering all possible point locations within a particular study region and to allow for edge effects in the geographic data retrieval for circles caused by a mixture of representational error (viz the use of 100 metre point references to represent postcodes and census enumeration districts of varying and different sizes and shapes) and locational inaccuracy (viz 100 metre point references instead of 1 metre references). The inclusion and exclusion of data points near the boundary of a circle may cause spurious patterns to appear. The overlaping circles offer a form of autosensitivity analysis that seemed to offer some advantages with this type of geographic data. This is a very important point that affects the use of spatial statistics. It is currently not known what effects this locational fuzziness has on many statistical methods, yet it is an endemic characteristic of geographic data sets. It is also a problem of growing magnitude because of the increasing use of GIS. However, it is recognised that because the circles overlap the resulting significance assessment for neighbouring circles is not necessarily independent. This defect is thought likely to make the GAM/1 a very sensitive pattern detector which may or may not be a desirable property depending on its propensity to produce false positives. On the other hand, it does at least attempt to incorporate geographic data uncertainty.

The spatial component of the generic hypothesis is easily handled. Having exhaustively evaluated all circles of a given radius, merely increase the radius a little, change the lattice spacing and thus the circle centroids, and then restart the analysis. This procedure is then repeated for a range of circle sizes; typically from 1km to 20km radii in instruments of 1km. It is not thought that the specification of these GAM search parameters will have a major effect on the results, provided their settings are not too coarse. This feeling is based on a number of computer runs but the effects remain to be quantified.

The final components in the GAM are the GIS and map display system. The former is necessary to allow point data to be efficiently retrieved for each of the million or so of circles of varying sizes. GAM/1 originally used a recursive tree based multi-path, multi-dimensional, data structure known as a KDB-tree. This allows the data to be stored on disk. Subsequently, GAM/1 has been reprogrammed for the Cray X_MP/48 at Rutherford and a simpler, less elegant, non-recursive but vectorizable bucket data structure was devised.

The reliance on the map as the final output from the GAM and as a visual representation of pattern may appear a little strange to non-geographers. However, it is quite acceptable to use a map based result evaluation system since GAM/1 was considered to be geo-descriptive technique. The eye-ball interpretation of map patterns may appear unscientific and arbitrary, but maps are very useful devices for communicating results and as a basis for further speculation about what patterns may or may not be present. At the same time the development of pattern recognition techniques have not yet been perfected to the extent that there is an automated alternative to the human eye-ball. It was conjectured that any dense, localised, concentration of circles that survive the significance assessment hurdle will provide a visual indication of spatial clustering. The ability to identify all areas within the study region where a null hypothesis appears to be breaking down is considered to be a very useful feature. It is also useful to be able to determine the full geographic extent of these patterns rather than restrict the analysis only on areas near observed cancer cases.

2.3 Running GAM/1

The GAM/1 has been run on preliminary cancer data for 0-15 year olds resident in Northern England at the time of diagnosis. All the data for a 1968-1985 time period is used for two disease categories; acute lymphoblastic leukaemia and Wilm's tumour. There is no time period or disease category permutation to be considered and no data disaggregation, although both would certainly be possible. The results have been reported in detail elsewhere (Openshaw et al., 1987, 1988) and will only be reviewed briefly. Figures 1 and 2 illustrate the type of patterns that emerge after computer run times of up to 6 hours on the Amdahl 5860 at Newcastle, using on this occasion an analytical Poisson calculation to assess significance. Although all the circles shown here have individual Poisson probabilities of less than 0.002, it is important to note that this is not the correct significance of the whole flock of circles occurring by chance. The significance testing procedure is used here purely as a benchmark for deciding which circles to plot.

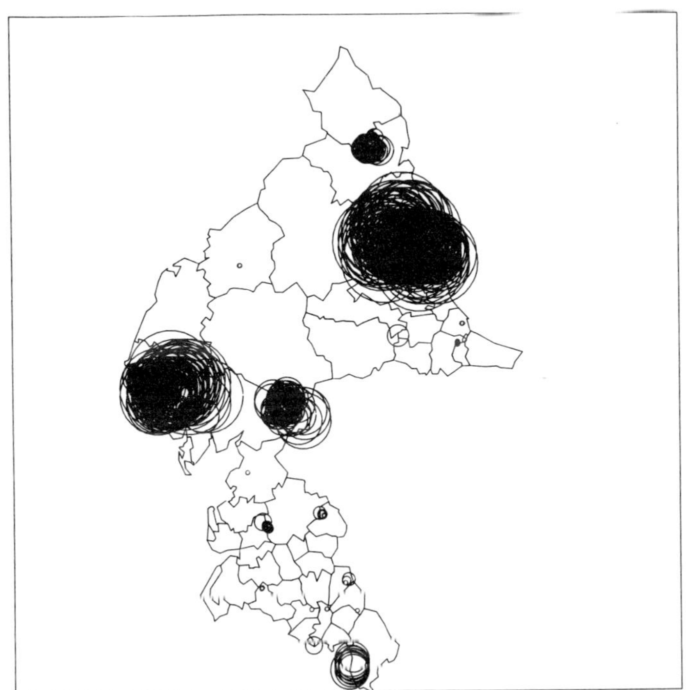

Fig. 1

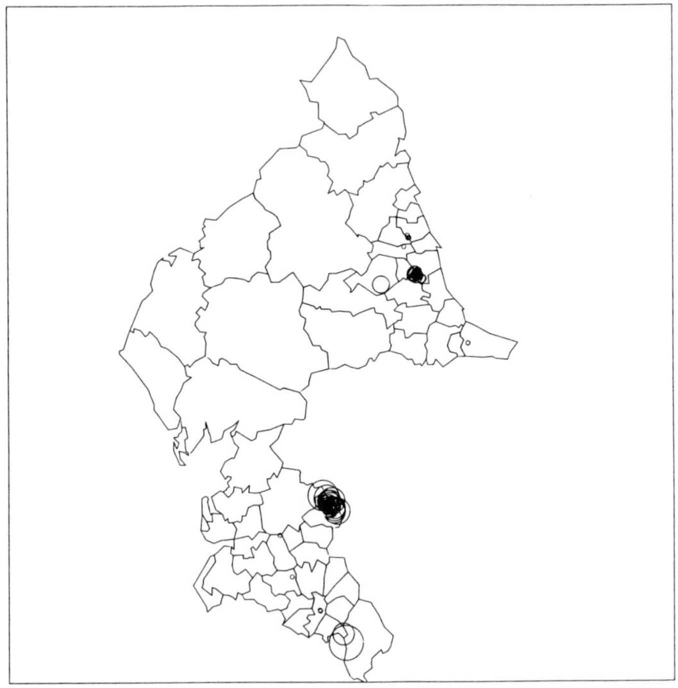

Fig. 2

The leukaemia results in Figure 1 show the expected Seascale cluster together with the even larger Gateshead-Tyneside cluster. The dense pattern of overlapping circles is formed by large numbers of individually "significant" circles, for a range of circle radii, concentrated together in close geographic proximity. These dense concentrations can be contrasted with qualitatively less dense flocks of circles which are of no great interest. By comparison, the Wilm's tumour data in Figure 2 contains little or no suggestion of clustering as very few individually significant circles are plotted. However, in both cases there is no means of knowing what is and what is not an interestingly dense concentration of significant circles.

The purpose in presenting these GAM/1 results is primarily descriptive. It offers a relatively unbiased view of those parts of the study region where there appears to be some evidence of spatial clustering, as witnessed by the presence of a large and seemingly unusual number of significant circles. The maps provide a framework that is informative and suggestive of further investigations. However, whether the patterns they contain are "real" and not chance occurrences can only be determined by further validation work involved simulation. Alternatively, an extension of the study region would be useful as a means of detecting recurrent patterns, which if they exist would offer a more substantive form of validation; for example, if a high percentage of clusters happened to be associated nationally with proximity to a particular land-use.

2.4 Some Problems With GAM/1

No technique is without limitations and GAM/1 is no exception. The emphasis placed on those problems thought to exist tends to reflect the statistical and to some extent philosophical standpoint of the inquirer. A list of problems would include;

(1) No measure of overall map pattern significance;

(2) The overlapping circles may result in too great a sensitivity to certain types of random pattern;

(3) There is no obvious way of comparing the map blobs formed by clusters of overlapping circles quantitatively;

(4) The power of its pattern detection abilities might well be different in urban compared with rural areas; and

(5) There is no satisfactory statistical basis for GAM/1.

These problems are not unexpected given the novel nature of the method and the underlying design objectives. Indeed, it is perhaps too easy to simply lose faith and dismiss the entire approach as being seductively attractive but fundamentally flawed, and then return to using more conventional methods which are equally flawed, but more widely accepted. There is no reason why these questions cannot be answered by simulation and, or, by developing GAM variants with different properties. There is also the danger of being over-cautious and too negative in dealing with new technology and by so doing denying access to potentially useful methods of analysis for no proven good reason. Clearly, some balanced and pragmatic decision is needed in a field where the public policy significance of the results strongly interacts with basic but as yet unanswered methodological questions. At what point you can go public with a new set of results is difficult to determine and any publication in such a sensitive area carries some risk. Under these circumstances caution is advised until there is evidence to substantiate either the results or more is known about the properties of the method. The use of the words "prototype" and "mark I" in the literature to describe the GAM/1 reflected these feelings and concerns.

3. VALIDATING THE GAM/1 RESULTS

One of the issues raised by the GAM/1 results in Figure 1 concerns the general high level of ignorance that exists regarding the nature of map patterns that purely random data might produce. A more pointed question concerns how often will "big blobs" appear in GAM/1 circle plots in purely random disease distributions? This is not a question that seemingly people have previously asked, yet it is clearly absolutely fundamental to the whole business of cluster detection. Without some assessment of the Type I error for the whole map pattern then there is no way of knowing precisely what the results mean. There are also other questions that need to be answered concerning the power of the procedure at detecting different types of pattern when pattern is known to exist, and vice versa. As it is more time consuming to answer this latter question, attention here is restricted to the former which is perhaps of more fundamental importance.

The procedure is fairly straightforward. First, run the GAM/1 499 times, an activity that would require approximately 5,000 hours of CPU time on the Amdahl 5860 at Newcastle University. Fortunately, there is a computationally more efficient alternative. The GAM/1 already has access to 499 random cancer distributions which were once used for an earlier Monte Carlo significance test based version. These random simulations reflect the distribution of the population at risk in 1981. It is a trival task to replace the Monte Carlo significance assessment by an analytical Poisson probability calculation, which yields very similar results. Then compute the analytical Poisson for each circle for each of the 499 random data sets in a single run and store all 500 sets of results. This reduced the computer run times to about two days for the acute lymphoblastic leukaemia data and about 10 hours for Wilm's tumour. Some guide as to likely whole map Type I errors can then be obtained by examining the GAM/1 results for these random data distributions.

Tables 1 and 2 show the top 10 ranked significant circle count data sets. The observed acute lymphoblastic data is ranked 5th out of the 500; the observed Wilm's data is ranked 168th. These results can be interpreted as implying that the approximate whole map Type I errors for the leukaemia data are about 5/500 and considerably higher, or 168/500 for Wilm's. Further qualitative insights can be gained by mapping the most densely circled random data GAM results. Figure 3 shows a selection of these top ranked random leukaemia maps. It is quite clear that it is possible to obtain one and sometimes two dense map blobs with random data, but that these are relatively rare. Eye-ball analysis would suggest a frequency of 10 out of 499, giving an approximate Type I error level of about 5%. However, nearly all these random data blobs appear in rural areas, and very few in urban areas. This is, of course, only to be expected since it only needs one or two cases to occur in an area low in children before significant circles appear, and provided the area is surrounded by other areas also deficient in children then the cluster will spread over a wide range of circle sizes. One conclusion is that, if anything, the Seascale cluster is less significant in this qualitative sense than the Gateshead-Tyneside one. Another is that a more automated blob detection technology is needed to firm up these subjective qualitative comparisons. High dimension maps which combine incidence and cancer counts might well provide a more useful way of looking at these patterns.

TABLE 1
TOP 10 RANKED "SIGNIFICANT" CIRCLE COUNT LEUKAEMIA DATA SETS

Rank	Simulation	Number of Significant Circles
1	491	1595
2	159	1403
3	259	1391
4	198	1387
5	Observed data	1357
6	283	1136
7	445	1036
8	447	1011
9	135	975
10	285	964

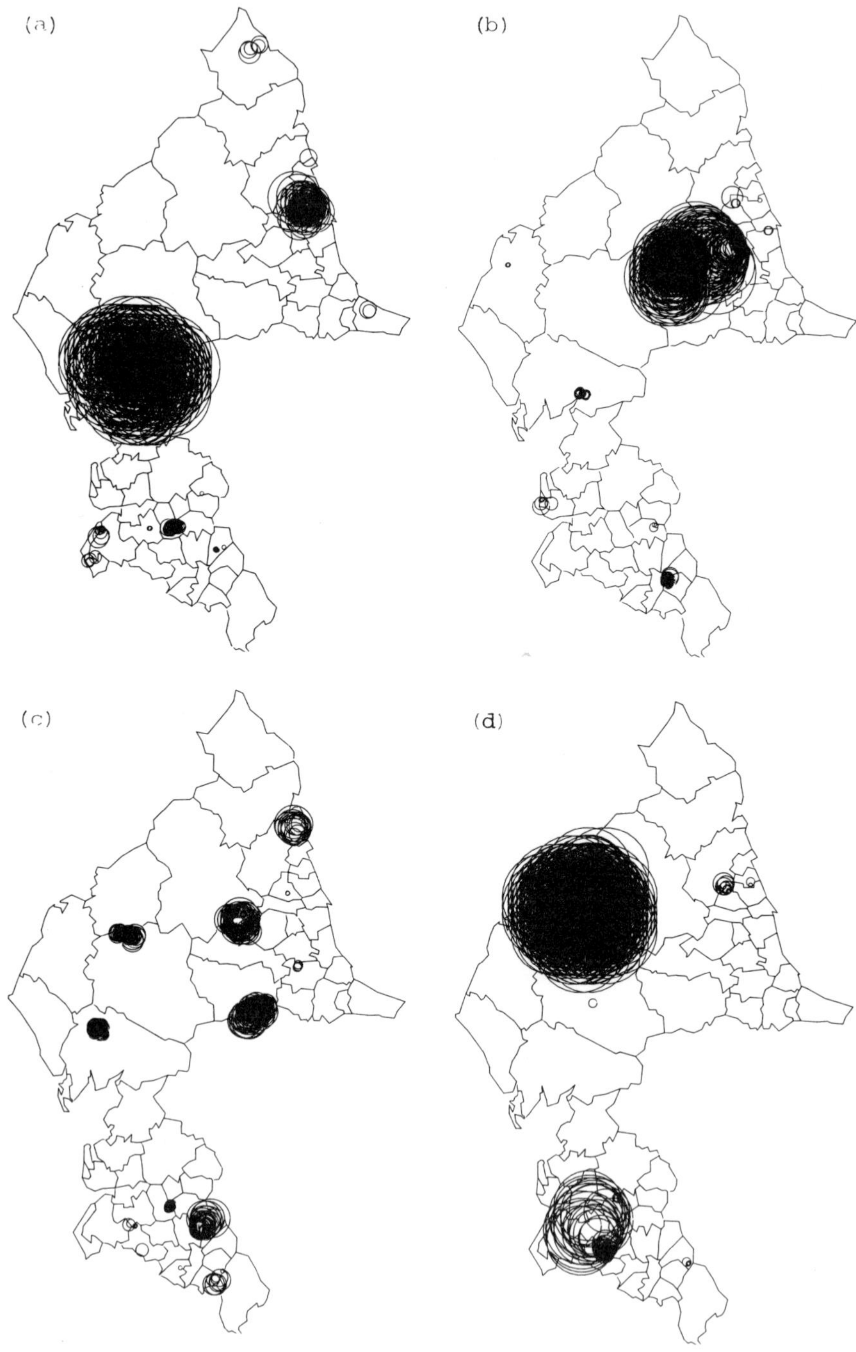

Fig. 3

TABLE 2
TOP 10 RANKED "SIGNIFICANT" CIRCLE COUNT WILMS DATA SETS

Rank	Simulation	Number of Significant Circles
1	259	882
2	35	734
3	174	693
4	2	686
5	8	672
6	283	672
7	310	667
8	96	658
9	348	643
10	350	639
168	Observed data	159

5. CONCLUSIONS

The paper has described an automated approach to the detection and validation of cancer clusters. It is argued that the rudimentary, mark I, geographical analysis machine does seem to work. Some very striking patterns have been identified that appear to be real rather than due to chance. However, clearly a considerable amount of further research and much more computer simulation will be needed before there is a complete understanding of what is going on. This includes understanding how the GAM interacts with any spatial patterns in the data and also investigating the impact of data shocks occasioned by the use of 1971 rather than 1981 population at risk information. The GAM/1 results almost certainly include a mix of both real and spurious circles and the task is how best to discriminate between them. However, the basic GAM technology is fairly flexible and can be presented in various guises; for example, based on a non-overlapping lattice or on circles designed to reach various population or cancer targets. Additionally, the pattern measuring and detection statistics can be changed; indeed, there is a number of potential spatial statistics that could be used instead of Poisson probabilities.

In evaluating these methods the provision of a standard set of synthetically generated "known pattern" benchmark data sets would be a useful means of evaluating new approaches in a comparable fashion. This also implies some common criteria for assessment and a standard measure of success. However, these academic concerns stand alongside intense medical interest in the results on real world data produced by techniques like GAM. Here the academic's caution gives way to a more pragmatic and real world concern with utilising whatever results are available in case they have some practical value.

The development of GAM has also served to emphasise the existence and importance of a whole string of interesting methodological problems, that are of course not all specific to the GAM techniques. Their resolution will take time, until then applications should proceed with care, emphasising the conditional nature of the results and the principle of caveat emptor. It is important to be at all times aware of both the specific limitations of a particular GAM and also the limitations of an exploratory style of study. All the GAM will do is provide evidence that clustering exists, whether it is due to socio-economic or demographic or migration effects should be discounted prior to any search for potential environmental causes. However, it is also important not to be too pessimistic. There is a feeling that if more applied mathematicians and statisticians were to be interested in this area, then the appropriate technology might be perfected sooner rather than later and the first generation methods based heavily on quantitative geographic technology could be replaced by second and third generation methods grounded more firmly, perhaps, in statistical and mathematical theory yet which are still able to take into account the endemic fuzziness of geographic data.

ACKNOWLEDGEMENTS

The author wishes to thank an ever lengthening list of people who have directly and indirectly contributed to this work. The data came from the two cancer registeries supported by the North of England Children's Cancer Research Fund and Cancer Research Campaign. Part of the GAM work was supported by the ESRC through their Northern Region Research Laboratory at Newcastle University. Finally, thanks are due to Alan Craft who started the whole GAM business by identifying the right question to ask.

REFERENCES

Openshaw, S., Charlton, M., Wymer, C. and Craft, A.W. (1987), A mark I geographical analysis machine for the automated analysis of point data sets, *International Journal of Geographic Information Systems*. 1, 335-358.

Openshaw, S., Charlton, M., Craft, A.W. and Birch, J.M. (1988), Investigation of leukaemia clusters by use of a geographical analysis machine, *The Lancet*, 272-273.

Wilkic, D. (1986), Transcript of Proceedings, Outline Planning Application for a European Demonstration Fast Reactor Reprocessing Plant at Dounreay, Caithness; Public Inquiry: Days 72-74, (mimeographed).

MODELLING THE SPREAD OF AIDS

J.D. Griffiths and K.A. Wheeler
(Department of Mathematics, UWIST, Cardiff)
*(Now: School of Mathematics,
University of Wales College of Cardiff)*

1. INTRODUCTION

Hardly a day passes without the media making some dire pronouncement regarding the AIDS (Acquired Immune Deficiency Syndrome) situation. Yet compared with the great pandemics of the past, AIDS would appear at first sight to be an insignificant disease. For example, the Spanish flu' epidemic, which swept through Europe in 1918, claimed over 20 million lives; compare this with a total of about 1350 AIDS cases and 750 deaths in the U.K. up to the end of March, 1988. Why then have the Government, and various other bodies, made such a drama of the AIDS problem? The answer to this question is many-fold. First and foremost, what we see at present is undoubtedly just the tip of the iceberg. If transmission of the Human Immunodeficiency Virus (HIV) ceased tomorrow, there would still be a considerable number of AIDS cases appearing for many years to come, since the disease has a long incubation period. It is estimated that there are between 50,000 and 100,000 virus carriers in the U.K. at the present time; many of these people are completely unaware that they are infected and hence may unwittingly pass the virus to others. Further cogent reasons for the concern being expressed in the various advertising campaigns are that AIDS tends to attack people in the prime of life, is invariably fatal, with death often occurring in a most unpleasant manner and above all the disease is preventable.

AIDS is thought to be a relatively new disease. The first cases were reported by the Centres for Disease Control (CDC) in Atlanta, U.S.A., in 1981, following recognition, by a number of astute physicians in several regions of America, of unexplained failure of the immune defence system in some of their patients. Once alerted to this new malady, reports quickly followed from other physicians in the U.S.A. and shortly afterwards from their counterparts in the U.K. and the rest of Europe. In 1983 the causative agent of the disease was found to be a virus. This was detected by French researchers under the direction of Luc Montangier at the Pasteur Institute in Paris, and independently by an American team under the leadership of Robert Gallo at the National Cancer Institute.

In 1982 CDC produced a case-definition of the conditions necessary for a person to be diagnosed as having AIDS. Basically, evidence is required of certain reliably diagnosed diseases which are indicative of an underlying cellular immune deficiency. In the U.K. approximately 65% of diagnoses list Pneumocystis Carinii Pneumonia as the indicative disease, while a further 23% of patients present with a rare form of skin cancer known as Kaposi's Sarcoma. Most of the remaining cases are diagnosed on the basis of certain other infections known as opportunistic infections.

The modes of transmission of the virus are now quite well understood, apart from one or two grey areas. The virus has been isolated from most body fluids, but in apparently varying concentrations. The most efficient means of transmission seems to be by blood-to-blood contact, and hence transfusions of infected blood or blood-products, the use of shared needles by Intravenous Drug Abusers, and certain homosexual practices have high risks associated with them.

2. ESTIMATING THE SPREAD OF AIDS INFECTION

Up to the end of March 1988, a total of 81,433 cases of AIDS from 133 countries had been reported to the World Health Organisation (WHO). Of these cases, 74% occurred in the Americas (66% in U.S.A., which has only 5% of the world population), 13% in Europe, 12% in Africa, and 1% in Asia. It seems certain that such figures disguise heavy under-reporting, particularly in Africa where resources for epidemiological studies are very limited. As conservative estimates of the true situation in 1987, WHO have suggested that there were 150,000 AIDS cases worldwide, and 5-10 million virus carriers. By 1991 WHO estimate that there will have been 2-3 million AIDS cases, and that 50-100 million persons will have been infected with the virus. Such estimates are a grim warning of the seriousness of the situation.

One needs to question the degree of accuracy and reliability which can be attached to estimates such as those quoted above. For example, are they based on the intuitive feelings of epidemiologists, or can they be substantiated by well-established statistical or mathematical techniques? It is quite clear that the potential magnitude of the problem makes it imperative, as far as allocation of resources, provision of medical and counselling care, etc is concerned, that estimates of the numbers of AIDS and HIV cases should be accurate and soundly based.

Many research groups in the U.K. and elsewhere in the world have produced models of varying degrees of complexity which purport to describe the spread of the AIDS epidemic, and of course each team tends to feel that their own model is the best under particular circumstances. At UWIST we have gone along a rather different path. Instead of concentrating on a particular model, we have investigated the potential usefulness of a number of different methods. Space restrictions do not allow detailed accounts of all the methods considered, but to fix ideas we will address the task of estimating the numbers of AIDS cases which will be apparent in the U.K. by the end of 1990.

The models considered are split into three categories: statistical projections, *ad hoc* methods, and mathematical models. Since the data required for input into sophisticated models is strictly limited, the emphasis has been on the use of simple models to provide order of magnitude estimates.

3. STATISTICAL PROJECTIONS

The basic data on which statistical estimates are founded are the numbers of AIDS cases reported each month. At once we are faced with a dilemma. Since AIDS is not a notifiable disease, it is highly likely that the number of cases reported does not represent a true picture of the situation. Should we therefore try to take account of this shortfall in some way, or should we predict on the basis of the reported data? In the absence of any reliable method of estimating the shortfall in reported cases, we have chosen to use the data as collected; at least this should provide a base line on which to work.

U.K. data is collected and summarised by the Communicable Diseases Surveillance Centre (CDSC) at Collingdale, and is reported monthly. Great care is taken to avoid errors, such as duplicate reporting, many of which are discovered retrospectively; this means that the data is in a continual state of flux, with alterations being made in data first reported months or even years previously.

The cumulative numbers of AIDS cases reported in the U.K. up to the end of 1987 are shown in Figure 1. The immediate impression gained from this diagram is one of exponential growth.

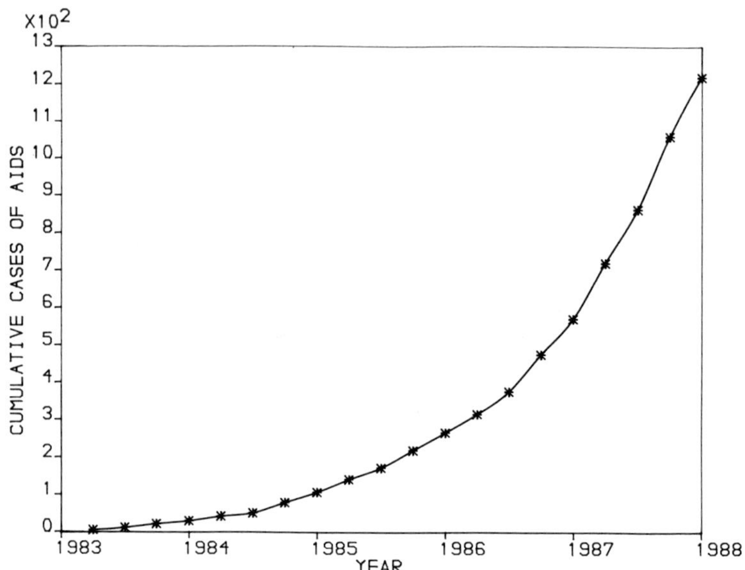

Fig. 1 Reported cases of AIDS to end of 1987

Suppose we postulate a simple model of the form

$$N(t) = N(o)\ e^{bt} \tag{3.1}$$

where N(t) is the total number of AIDS cases reported by time t, b is a constant, and t is measured from the beginning of 1983 (when records began).

Thus, if the assumption of exponential growth is justified, we might expect that an approximately linear relationship would be apparent from plotting log N(t) against t. Figure 2 shows such a plot with the least squares line fitted. It is clear to the naked eye, without recourse to statistical confirmation, that a straight line is not the most appropriate curve to fit. The extrapolated value for the cumulative number of AIDS cases at the end of 1990 is 41,880.

If we fit a model of the form $\log N(t) = ct^d$ to the data shown in Figure 2, then the least squares values of c and d are

$$c = 0.736, \quad d = 0.480$$

This produces a value of 7800 for the cumulative number of AIDS cases by 1990 - vastly different from the straightforward log-linear fit.

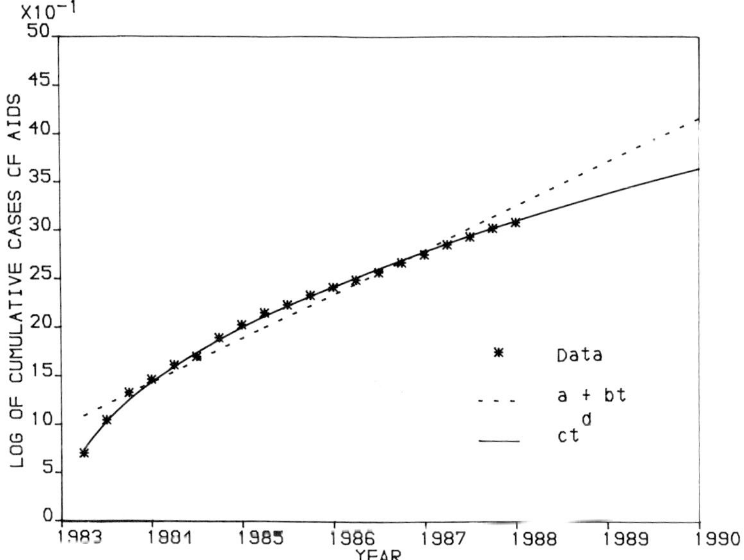

Fig. 2 Log-linear fit to cumulative reported cases of AIDS

It is also possible to use techniques similar to those outlined above on the numbers of new cases reported in specified time intervals (for example, each quarter). The previous notation needs some modification. Let

$$n(i) = ge^{hi} \qquad i = 1,2, \ldots\ldots$$

where n(i) is the number of new cases reported in the i'th quarter, and g, h are constants.

Again one would expect a linear association between log n(i) and i if this model is to be appropriate. Figure 3 shows this data together with the least squares line. In this case the straight line fit is at least believable. The least squares equation gives

$$n(i) = 3.855\ e^{0.207i}$$

with correlation coefficient 0.97

Using this method the predictions for the numbers of new cases in 1988, 1989, 1990 are 1670, 3820, 8740 respectively, giving a total of 15,460 by the end of 1990. The confidence limits on this latter figure are very wide, 9900 - 24700.

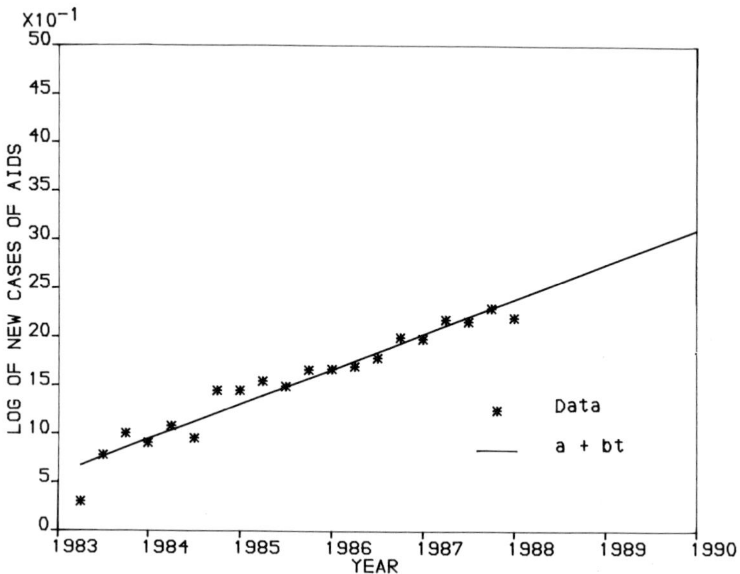

Fig. 3 Log-linear fit to new reported cases of AIDS

A measure of the severity of the epidemic which receives much media attention is the so-called doubling time. In essence this provides the same information as a regression approach but in a rather more digestible form. If we first consider the cumulative number of cases of AIDS at any instant, the doubling time is the period required to see that number of cases double. Using the simple model proposed by (3.1) it is easy to show that the doubling time is given by ln 2/b, where b is the regression coefficient in the log-linear fit. Inspection of Figure 1 indicates that in fact the doubling time is not constant. For example in 1983 it was about 6 months, whereas in 1986 it has increased to about 10 months. This indicates that a rather different approach from traditional regression analysis is required. We could undertake log-linear fits over short periods of time (called windows), in essence providing a series of piece-wise regressions. Windows would typically be of length two or three years. A series of such window-length regressions would produce corresponding values of b, which could then be translated into doubling times. Although the authors have undertaken such analyses, the labour involved is hardly worth the effort. Much the same results are obtained by taking the cumulative number of cases at the end of any year, and then using Figure 1 (or an equivalent algebraic approach) to find how many months elapse before this number doubles. Table 1 gives the doubling times (in months) for each of the years 1982-1986. We may then project the trend in these doubling times using the curve fitting techniques for cumulative cases outlined earlier. Using a fairly straightforward inversion process we may convert these doubling times to cumulative cases of AIDS. The results are given in Table 2. Again we may do slightly better by using a non-linear fit. The projection yields 7960 cases by 1990.

A similar exercise may be undertaken using the numbers of new cases of AIDS reported per quarter. In this instance the doubling time is the period taken before a quarter appears with twice the initial number of new cases.

Doubling Time for Cumulative Number of Cases of AIDS

End of half year		Actual Doubling Time (months)
1982	2	3.5
1983	1	3.4
	2	6.9
1984	1	5.4
	2	8.5
1985	1	10.8
	2	10.8
1986	1	10.7
	2	10.0

Table 1

DOUBLING TIME FOR CUMULATIVE NUMBER OF CASES OF AIDS

Year end	Actual Doubling Time (months)	Predicted Doubling times (months)			
		DT=a+bx	cum cases	DT=ax^b	cum cases
1982	3.5				
1983	6.9				
1984	8.5				
1985	10.8				
1986	10.0				
1987		13.9	1256	12.8	1256
1988		16.0	2340	14.2	2433
1989		18.0	4095	15.5	4489
1990		20.0	6825	16.7	7964

Table 2

4. AD HOC METHODS

Within this category we shall include methods which do not have a direct statistical or modelling connotation.

It is clear from the data given earlier that the spread of AIDS in the U.S.A. is of a different magnitude to that reported elsewhere in the world. It would seem sensible therefore to attempt to gain insight from the American experience.

Up to the end of 1987 there were 51,361 AIDS cases reported in the U.S.A.; in comparison the number of U.K. cases reported was 1227. If one searches through the American data to discover when their cumulative total was 1227 cases we find that this occurred in early 1983, a lag of 4.7 years. However a moment's reflection indicates that this is not a fair means of comparison; the population of the two countries differs by a factor of about 4. A more meaningful comparison is given in Figure 4, where the numbers of cases per million population are shown. It can be seen that in the early stages of the epidemic the lag in incidence was about 2.5 years; at the end of 1987 it had increased to 3.5 years. Thus to predict the cumulative total of U.K. cases at the end of 1990, we need the U.S.A. incidence at mid-1987. This was 147.3 cases per million inhabitants. Applying this incidence to a U.K. population of 56 million produces a cumulative total of 8250 AIDS cases. It may be possible to make the estimation procedure a little more accurate, since it appears that the lag in incidence is not constant. We might postulate that by the end of 1990 the lag will have increased to 4.5 years. This converts to an estimate of about 6000 U.K. cases by December, 1990.

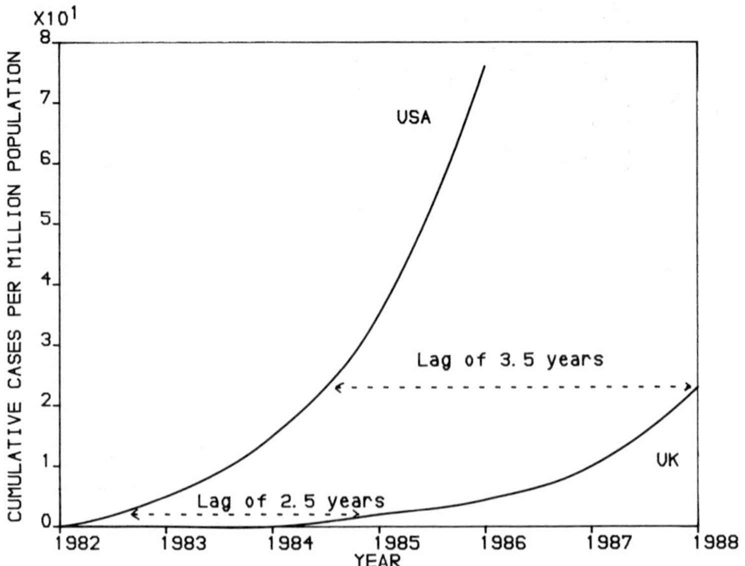

Fig. 4 Incidence of AIDS in USA and UK

We now turn to a completely different method of estimation. It is a sad fact that most of the persons who will be diagnosed as having AIDS in the intervening years to 1990 are already infected with the virus. The *incubation period* is defined as the interval of time elapsing between infection with the virus and the onset of full-blown AIDS. The date of diagnosis of AIDS in a patient is a good indicator of the onset of the disease. Unfortunately it is not easy in the majority of cases to establish when infection took place; for example, transmission via homosexual acts could occur from any of a number of contacts spread over a considerable period of time. However there is a set of data from which it is possible to estimate the date of infection quite precisely, see Peterman, et al. (1985). These data refer to AIDS patients in the U.S.A. who received a single transfusion of infected blood or blood products. All other likely causes of infection with HIV were eliminated from 297 such AIDS cases. Medley, et al (1987) found that a Weibull distribution produced a good fit to the distribution of incubation times. The two-parameter Weibull distribution has the density function

$$f(x) = pq^p x^{p-1} e^{-(qx)^p} \qquad x \geqslant 0$$

where p and q are the parameters to be determined. Using maximum likelihood techniques, the fitted parameter values are p = 2.396, q = 0.1077 for adult cases in the age range 5-59 years, giving a mean and median incubation period of 8.23 and 7.97 years respectively. The values of the parameters are very different for the age range 0-4 years, but there are far fewer cases of AIDS/HIV infection in this age group, and we shall concentrate our argument on adult cases.

Suppose we make the assumption that the doubling time of HIV infection is similar to that of AIDS, and that 1 infective was introduced to the UK sometime during 1980. Table 3 gives the results of a possible scenario. Using the assumed doubling times we can estimate the cumulative numbers of HIV positive cases for each year, and hence deduce the number of new HIV positives occurring in each year. Using the percentage points of the cumulative Weibull distribution we can then estimate the number of AIDS cases by the end of 1990 which stem from each of the earlier years' HIV cases. This gives a cumulative total of 19750 by the end of 1990. However, there is some belief that only 50% - 75% of HIV positives will ever develop full-blown AIDS. Using this assumption the prediction for 1990 gives a cumulative total of AIDS cases in the range 9880 - 14810.

Weibull Distribution fitted to Incubation Period

Onset Year	Doubling Time (months)	Cumulative no. infected by end of year	No. Infected during the year	Weibull Distribution Proportion	AIDS cases by end 1990
1980	3				
1981	3	4		.70	3
1982	3	64	60	.61	37
1983	6	1,024	960	.50	480
1984	6	4,096	3,072	.40	1,229
1985	12	16,384	12,288	.30	3,686
1986	12	32,768	16,384	.20	3,277
1987	12	65,536	32,768	.12	3,932
1988	18	131,072	65,536	.064	4,194
1989	18	218,453	87,381	.025	2,185
1990	18	364,088	145,635	.005	728

Total Cumulative Cases of AIDS by 1990 = 19,751

Table 3

5. A MATHEMATICAL MODEL

One of the advantages of a mathematical model is that it is possible to interrogate the system on the familiar "what if?" basis. Another advantage, in comparison with statistical projections which merely extrapolate supposed trends, is that it is possible to build whatever knowledge exists relating to factors such as transmission mechanisms, incubation periods, etc., into mathematical models.

Inspection of data from CDSC shows that about 85% of reported AIDS cases in the UK may be linked to homosexual transmission, and it seems reasonable therefore to attempt to model cases resulting from this particular transmission characteristic.

Consider the group of sexually active homosexuals in the UK. By 'sexually active' we shall mean homosexuals who indulge in 'high risk' behaviour. 'Non-sexually active' will be taken to mean no involvement in high risk behaviour. We assume the group may be divided into three subgroups:

(i) *Susceptibles* - those not yet infected with the virus,

(ii) *Infectives* - those infected with HIV but not yet diagnosed as having AIDS

(iii) *AIDS* - those diagnosed as having full-blown AIDS.

Figure 5 gives a diagrammatic representation of the model. We introduce the following notation. At time t, let

$X(t)$ be the number of sexually active susceptibles,

$Y(t)$ be the number of sexually active HIV positives,

$V(t)$ be the number of non-sexually active HIV positives,

$A(t)$ be the number of sexually active AIDS patients.

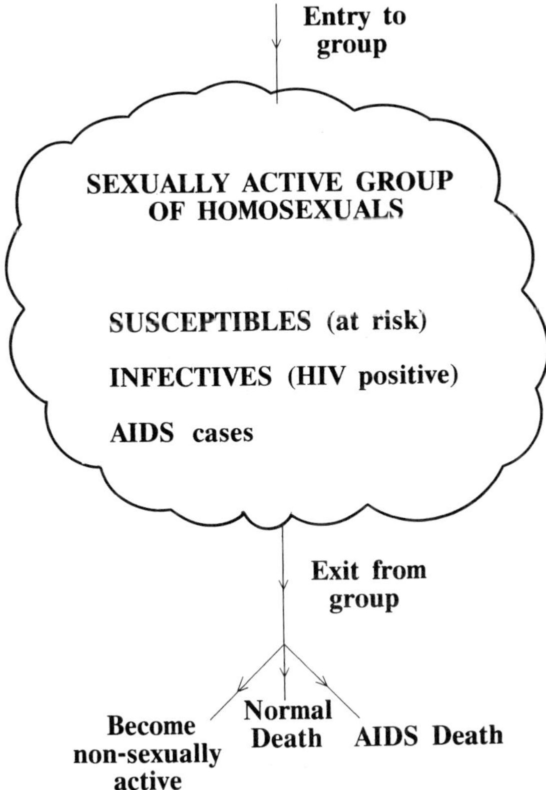

Fig. 5 Diagrammatic representation of mathematical model

Figure 6 shows a flow diagram illustrating possible transition paths. The parameters ν_i (i = 1,2,3,) represent the rate at which individuals in the various groups change from sexually active to non-active (perhaps through fear, or as a result of education campaigns); the parameters μ_i (i = 1,2,3) represent 'normal' death rates (i.e. deaths from causes other than AIDS); ω indicates the death rate from AIDS. The parameter α represents the rate at which susceptibles become infected with HIV; it is assumed that a proportion of these, a, continue to be sexually active (they may not know that they are infected), while the remainder become non-sexually active. We assume that the transition rate from HIV positive to full-blown AIDS is γ, with a proportion, b, of those infectives who were previously sexually active remaining so and a proportion, g, of those infectives who were not sexually active previously now becoming active.

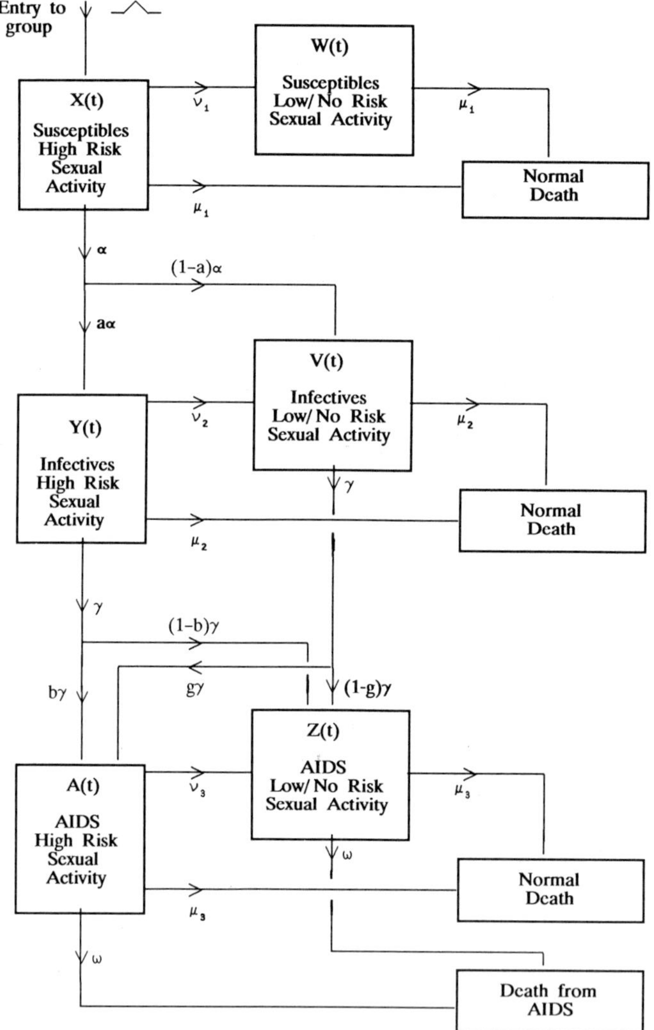

Fig. 6 Flow diagram for mathematical model

The infection rate α requires further explanation. It would seem reasonable to assume that the chance of infection is proportional to the number of different sexual partners a susceptible has, and also to the probability that a partner is infected. The number of infected sexually active homosexuals at any time is $Y(t) + A(t)$, and hence the probability that a partner chosen at random from the population is infected is $[Y(t) + A(t)]/N(t)$, where $N(t) = X(t) + Y(t) + A(t)$. Thus

$$\alpha = \beta c[Y(t) + A(t)]/N(t)$$

where c is the mean number of sexual partners a homosexual has, and β is a constant.

Using Figure 6 it is a fairly straightforward task to set up the following differential equations

$$\frac{dX}{dt} = \mu_1 N(t) - (\nu_1 + \mu_1)\, X(t) - \frac{\beta c}{N(t)}[Y(t) + A(t)]\, X(t)$$

$$\frac{dY}{dt} = \frac{a\,\beta c}{N(t)}[Y(t) + A(t)]\, X(t) - (\nu_2 + \mu_2 + \gamma)\, Y(t)$$

$$\frac{dV}{dt} = \nu_2\, Y(t) + \frac{(1-a)\beta c\, X(t)}{N(t)}[Y(t) + A(t)] - (\mu_2 + \gamma)\, V(t)$$

$$\frac{dA}{dt} = b\,\gamma\, Y(t) + g\,\gamma\, V(t) - (\mu_3 + \nu_3 + \omega)\, A(t)$$

Analytic solution of these four non-linear equations seems improbable. However the equations yield readily to numerical solution. The parameter values used in the analysis are as follows (all rates are per year):

$\nu_1 = 0.1$, $\nu_2 = 0.1$, $\nu_3 = 0.5$

$\mu_1 = 0.031$, $\mu_2 = 0.031$, $\mu_3 = 0.031$, $\omega = 1$

$a = 0.9$, $b = .5$, $g = 0.1$

$\beta c = 0.957$ $\gamma = 0.02$, $N(o) = 10^6$

Space restrictions do not permit detailed arguments for the choice of these parameter values.

Figure 7 provides a comparison of the cumulative numbers of reported AIDS cases to the end of 1987 with those predicted by the model. An interesting side issue resulting from this analysis is that by extrapolating backwards, the first HIV infection in the UK would have taken place as early as 1973 - a view now held by many clinicians.

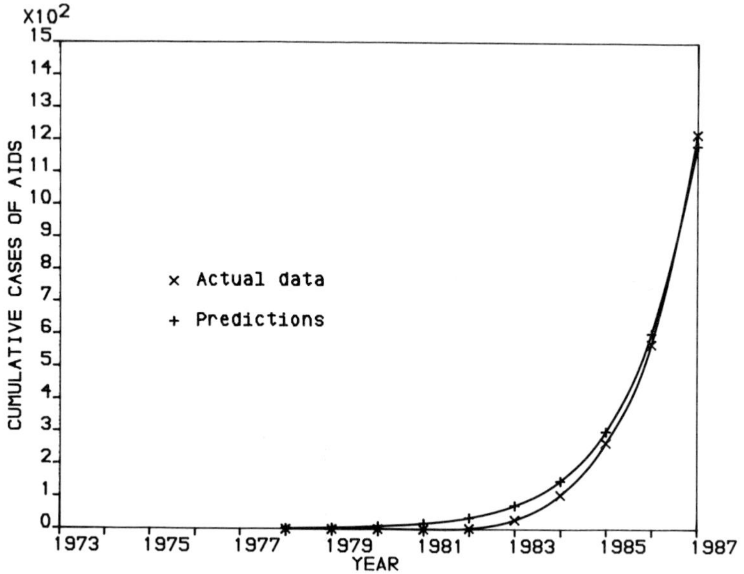

Fig. 7 Comparison between model predictions and reported cases of AIDS

Figure 8 shows the development of new cases of AIDS over the next forty years. It can be seen that new cases reach a peak in the mid-1990's with about 3,500 cases per year being reported. The estimate for the cumulative number of cases by the end of 1990 is 6,380.

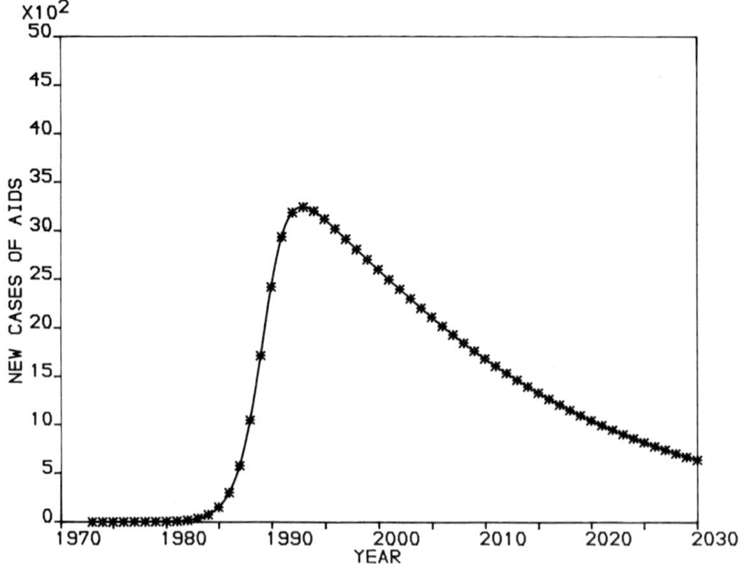

Fig. 8 Model predictions of new cases of AIDS to year 2030

We now use the model to investigate various intervention effects. Suppose a vaccine became available which could prevent susceptibles becoming infected with HIV (we assume that such a vaccine has no benefit to those already infected). If such a vaccine were introduced in 1988, then the effect would be quite dramatic, as shown in Figure 9. However it seems unlikely that such a vaccine will be developed for some years. If we consider introduction of the vaccine in 1993, Figure 9 shows that the reduction in cumulative cases of AIDS is quite small. This result is interesting since it raises policy decisions relating to the advisability of spending scarce resources on development of vaccines.

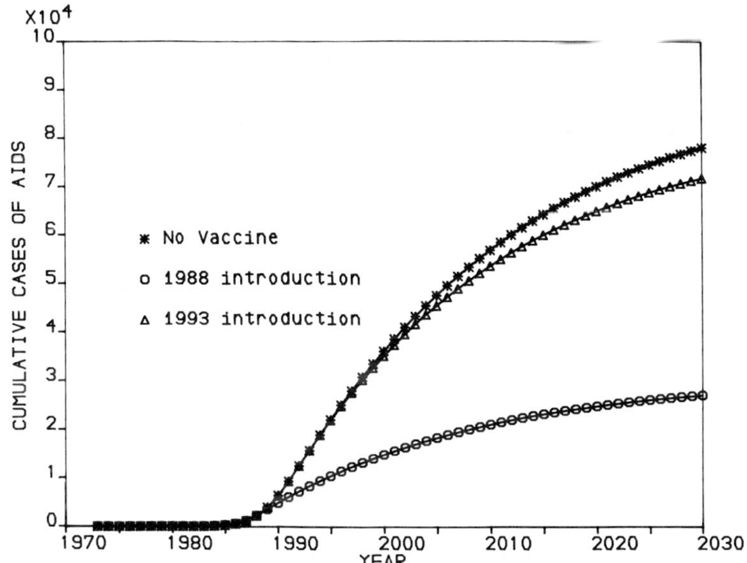

Fig. 9 Effect of introducing vaccine for susceptibles

Suppose now that a drug is produced which would prevent those infected with HIV from developing AIDS. (It is assumed that drug, unlike a vaccine, would not prevent susceptibles from becoming infected). Since such drugs are likely to be expensive, and could have undesirable side-effects, it is pertinent to consider the effect of giving the drug to only a proportion of the infected population. Figure 10 shows the effects of the introduction of such a drug in 1993 when it is made available, on the one hand to the total infected population and on the other hand to only 10% of those infected. It can be seen that unless quite high coverage is ensured, the savings in AIDS cases would be small. The difficulties associated with achieving a high take-up rate for this type of drug must be borne in mind, since a large proportion of the HIV positive population are completely unaware that they are infected.

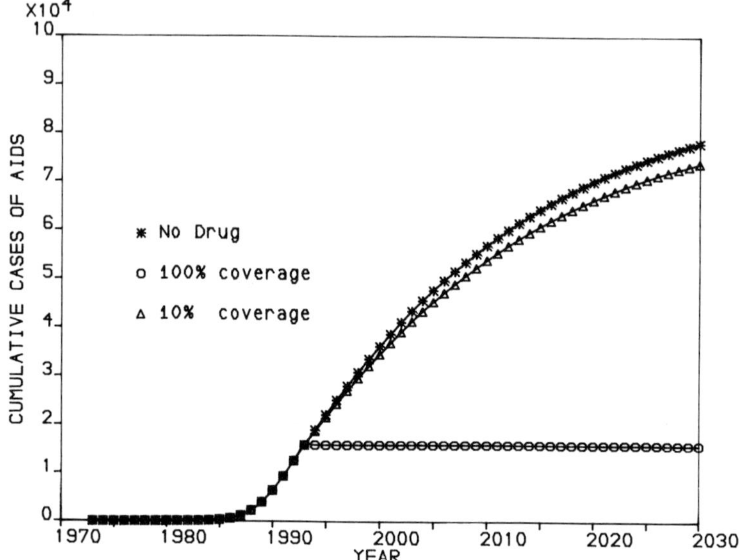

Fig. 10 Effect of introducing drug to prevent infecteds from developing AIDS

Finally we look at possible effects of the education campaigns. Suppose that these result in reducing c, the mean number of sexual partners which a homosexual has. Figure 11 shows the number of AIDS cases for reductions in c in 1988 to 10%, 50%, 90% of its previously assumed value. It can be seen that substantial changes in behaviour are needed before any dramatic fall-off in AIDS cases is noticed.

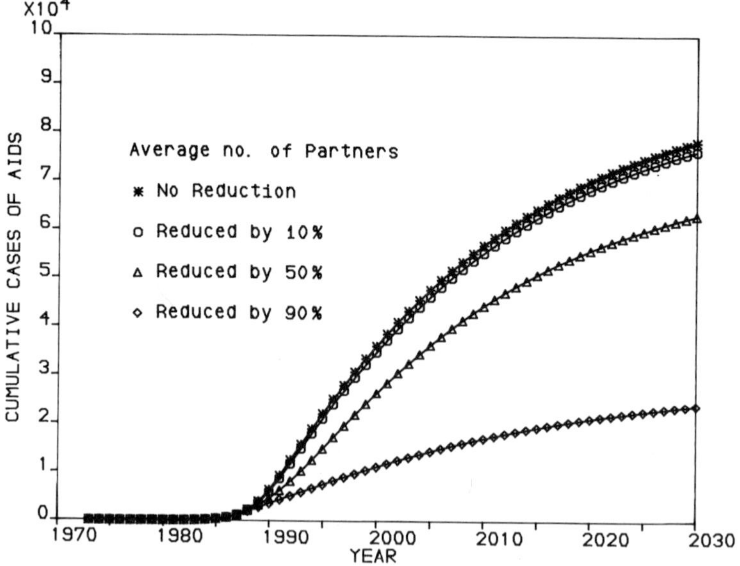

Fig. 11 Effect of reduction in numbers of sexual partners

6. SUMMARY

As stated in section 2, the objective of this paper was to estimate the cumulative number of AIDS cases in the UK by the end of 1990. This task has been undertaken using a variety of statistical and mathematical methods; the projections are based on data existing at the end of 1987.

Table 4 summarises the results of this exercise. It is immediately apparent that the table has one extreme outlying estimate - that provided by log-linear regression on cumulative cases. The explanation as to why it is unwise to use this method (even for the modest 3-year extrapolation in this case) has been given in section 3. The log-linear regression on new cases of AIDS also gives a rather high estimate, thus giving some credence to the belief that exponential growth models are no longer appropriate at this stage of the epidemic.

SUMMARY OF RESULTS

Method	Estimated Cumulative Cases of AIDS at end of 1990
Log Linear Regression on Cumulative Cases	41,880
Power index Regression on Cumulative Cases	7,800
Log Linear Regression on New Cases	15,460
Linear Regression on Doubling Times	6,830
Power index Regression on Doubling Times	7,960
USA v UK Lag	8,250
Incubation period	9,800 - 14,810
UWIST Mathematical Model	6,380
Inst. of Actuaries' Model	8,420 - 10,580

Table 4

The remaining estimates cluster around the 8,000 mark - it should be remembered that the objective was to produce an order of magnitude projection - with the UWIST mathematical model producing the lowest estimate. It is interesting to reflect that by the time this paper appears in print much of the data referring to the period up to 1990 will be available. The proof of the pudding is in the eating!

7. REFERENCES

Peterman, T.A., Drotman, D.P. and Curran, J.W., (1985) Epidemiology of the Acquired Immunodeficiency Syndrome (AIDS), Epidemiologic Reviews, 7, 1-21.

Peterman, T.A., Jaffe, H.W., Feorino, P.M., Getchell, J.P., Warfield, D., Haverkos, H.W., Stoneburner, R.L. and Curran, J.W., (1985) Transfusion-associated Acquired Immunodeficiency Syndrome in the United States. *J.A.M.A.* 254, 2913-2917.

Medley, G.F., Anderson, R.M., Cox, D.R. and Billard, L., (1987) Incubation period of AIDS in patients infected via blood transfusion, Nature 6132, 719-721.

THE IDENTIFICATION AND INVESTIGATION OF EPIDEMICS

S. R. Palmer
*(Public Health Laboratory Service
Regional Epidemiologist for Wales)*

This paper is intended to provide an insight into the practical aspects of outbreak investigation and the way in which statistical methods are used in field epidemiology as well as their limitations.

The classical approach to infectious disease epidemiology is the detailed investigation of individual cases in the light of the well established microbiological features of the particular infection and a confidence in the possible routes of transmission. Descriptive data is then analysed by the three classical parameters of time, place and person. This "shoe leather" approach can be illustrated by an outbreak of *Salmonella paratyphi* infection in the UK. This particular infection is very rarely acquired within the UK and the occurrence of just three cases who had not travelled overseas within the incubation period of the infection warranted urgent investigation. On 23/6/86 a 14 year old girl became ill with abdominal pain and watery diarrhoea and fever. A blood culture was positive for *S. paratyphi B* phage type dundee. On 10/10/86 a 14 year old boy from the same school but a different form, living within half a mile of case 1, developed fever, rigors, headache and flu-like symptoms which was followed 3 days later by diarrhoea. A faeces sample taken on 22/10/86 was positive for *S.paratyphi B* phage type dundee. Case 2 did not have close contact with case 1. Neither had travelled outside of the town in the four weeks before onset. On 26/10/86 a 70 year old woman living in the same neighbourhood as cases 1 and 2 became ill with nausea, fever, giddiness and abdominal pain and was admitted to hospital on 2/11/86 dehydrated and confused. A urine sample taken on 7/11/86 yielded *S. paratyphi B* phage type dundee. Interviews with cases 1-3 revealed two common food suppliers used in the month before onset, a supermarket and a local fish and chip shop. Cases 1 and 2 had eaten fish and chips from there regularly but case 3 bought fish and chips on only one occasion three weeks before onset of illness. The shop was visited by an Environmental Health Officer and it was discovered that the proprietor had been admitted to the local hospital in 1980 with S. paratyphi B infection on return from holiday in Egypt. Laboratory records at the hospital were reviewed and the organism was confirmed to have been S. paratyphi B phage type dundee. In March 1986 three months before illness in the first case he purchased the fish and chip shop. Faeces samples were obtained from the proprietor who was positive. Almost certainly, in this outbreak the three cases acquired infection from eating contaminated food handled by the proprietor. The evidence was considered sufficient to put the proprietor off work immediately. S. paratyphi B carriage is very unusual in the UK, the organism is known to be a food borne infection and chronic carriage leading to contamination of food and subsequent transmission of infection is well documented.

Descriptive data in the absence of microbiological confirmation however are not always a sufficient basis for introducing control measures. Caution is needed in the analysis and interpretation of data from cases, especially data about place and person. For example, in an outbreak of Salmonella paratyphi B phage type 3a var 4 extending over 4 years which exclusively affected holidaymakers visiting Portugal all cases except the last 3 had eaten at one restaurant in one small village. This restaurant had therefore been considered the most likely source of infection for the first three years, although screening of food handlers failed to identify a carrier. However, when local data were eventually obtained it was found that the particular restaurant was the only one sited on the resort beach and that most if not all visitors would eat at the restaurant. The last three cases visited the resort after the restaurant had closed for the season. The probably source of infection was found to be raw sewage which was contaminating the beach from a faulty sewer drain. Thus, observations on the cases have to be set against what is expected in the population from which they come: in the example above, all holidaymakers visiting the resort would be expected to eat at the restaurant.

Descriptive data may suggest hypotheses to be tested by analytical methods. Broadly there are two complementary approaches the microbiological, eg. culturing foods remaining from a meal thought to have caused food poisoning and the epidemiological. Even when microbiological investigations reveal contamination (e.g. legionellae in a hospital cooling tower) this does not in itself identify the source of infection. Epidemiological evidence is still necessary to demonstrate an association between, for example, the cooling tower drift and the occurrence of illness. Since most water stored in large buildings will yield legionellae, but outbreaks are relatively rare, the significance of environmental isolates will need to be determined epidemiologically.

Essentially the epidemiological approach is to compare the characteristics of infected persons (cases) with those of a similar group of uninfected persons (controls). Two principal study designs are used, the case-control and the cohort study. In both cases microbiological data is crucial to correct interpretation. For example, an outbreak of Salmonella typhimurium in a university hostel affected 66 students (1). A questionnaire survey of all residents in the hall recorded symptoms, date of onset of illness and foods consumed. However, calculation of food specific attack rates did not reveal an association with any particular food item. In this investigation stool samples were obtained from well persons as well as cases. Sixteen of 180 symptomless students were faeces positive. Twelve of 65 symptomatic students were faeces negative and may have been suffering from other illnesses. Only when cases were defined by positive faeces samples did a statistically significant difference in attack rates for different foods consumed emerge. This outbreak investigation emphasises the need for precise microbiological definition of a case and the need to minimise misclassification of symptomless but infected individuals.

In some outbreaks, however, the descriptive epidemiology suggests hypotheses which go against the accepted microbiological theory. For example, Shingles is considered to result from the reactivation of latent varicella zoster (VZ) virus which has survived in sensory ganglia following chickenpox in childhood. Susceptible people may contract chickenpox from patients with shingles but it is usually said that the reverse process does not occur. However a cluster of cases of shingles occurred in workers at the DVLC with features strongly suggestive of direct person to person transmission (2). Between May and August 1983 7 employees working in one department contracted shingles. Serological tests confirmed the diagnosis of recent varicella activity. The incidence of doctor-certificated shingles in the whole workforce and in a control population was calculated from personnel records. Associations between cases and place of work in the index department were examined from the records of assigned weekly work areas. The environment of the workplace was examined for toxic or other possible environmental causes of immunosuppression. No sources of radiation were present and none of the chemical compounds used in the workplace were known to be associated with shingles or other infections. In 1983 there were 26 cases of GP certificated shingles in the 4165 workforce but 7 of these were in the 101 employees in the index department $\psi^2 = 59.8$, $p < 10^{-11}$). Applying age specific incidence rates observed in the rest of the workforce to the index department gave expected numbers of women and men cases of 0.55 and 0.12 respectively, compared with the observed 5 and 2. The probability of observing 6 or more cases in one month among 101 employees was calculated using the Poisson distribution and the overall 1983 incidence of 26 cases per 4165 employees; it was 3×10^{-11}. This figure is based on the assumption that cases occur at random with equal chance among all employees and it has been shown that risk of shingles increases with age. However 5 of the 6 cases which occurred within 1 month were aged over 40 years. The monthly incidence rate of those over 40 years in the total workforce was 1.04/1000 and the chance of observing 5 or more cases in 62 employees would be 1×10^{-8}. If the statistical analysis is limited to within the index department there is evidence of clustering in time. Using exact probabilities and considering 1983 as 6 two-month periods the chance of observing 6 of the 7 cases in July and August if cases occurred at random is 0.0008.

In addition to the statistical evidence of clustering there was evidence of close contact between cases which might represent a chain of transmission. The index department comprised an open floor area on one side of which were enclosed offices and the sequence of onsets of shingles was related to the proximity to a prior case with an incubation period of about 10 days. All 5 cases who were machine operators worked in two adjacent units but only 2 of the 9 matched controls worked in these units over the same "exposure" periods (exact two tailed probability = 0.006).

Shingles is universally regarded as the reactivation of latent VZ virus infection and therefore would not be expected to present in outbreaks due to person to person transmission of virus. The causes of reactivation of latent VZ virus are not well described although the elderly and the immunosuppressed are more at risk. We suggested from the evidence of this outbreak that re-exposure to varicella virus may provoke the recrudescence of latent endogenous virus leading to shingles.

The interpretation of the cluster of cases has been challenged on the basis that by chance a cluster of shingles cases would be expected in a group of 100 people somewhere in the world every 36 months (3). On the basis of statistical probabilities calculated on the outbreak data no definitive answer to this can be given (4). Clearly, the cluster was an unlikely event but was it purely a chance coincidence? The descriptive data showing a pattern resembling person to person transmission is the strongest indication that currently accepted dogma about the aetiology of shingles may be incomplete.

The difficulty of interpreting statistically significant associations in the absence of a plausible mechanism of causation is further illustrated by the following example. Given the lack of knowledge about the causes of aplastic anaemia, a life threatening disease, the occurrence of a cluster of three cases presenting to one hospital over a 2 week period led to a detailed investigation of possible environmental causes (4). No chemicals, commercial products, or medicines, were used by all three patients or kept in the homes of all three families. None of the three had a history of significant exposure to chemicals. The three cases did not know each other and had not met before hospital admission. One possible environmental exposure was suggested by the finding that all three patients visited the same swimming pool and the surrounding area over a short period. This was an unexpected finding since the particular pool was on the opposite side of the city to the cases. In case 1 who lived 15 miles to the West of the city the only visit to the city in the 6 months prior to onset was to this swimming pool and to a family friend who lived nearby. Case 2 also visited the same pool on 2 or 3 occasions at about the same period and also visited his grandparents who lived in the same road as the family friends of case 1. Case 3 whilst living in the far West of the city went to school on the East, near to the swimming pool and used the pool during school sessions. His school bus stop was in the road where the other patients visited, and was only a few yards from these houses. Detailed enquiries were made with the swimming pool authorities and with the Parks department of the Local Authority. Pool maintenance was satisfactory and there was no record of unusual chemicals being used in the pool, nor of accidents with chemicals. There was no record of chemicals being spilled in the vicinity and the weedkiller used by the Local Authority for the roadside in April was also used throughout the city.

Two opposite approaches were taken to this cluster. The field epidemiologist interpreted the pattern of occurrence as suggesting the existence of a common factor in the environment which should be investigated and identified urgently to prevent further cases. An academic epidemiologist considered that in the absence of a known aetiology for aplastic anaemia the cluster was due to chance. The implications for allocation of public health field work resources was significant. The argument might be put forward that any three people questioned in depth would turn out to have at least one common time/place exposure. On the other hand experience of interviewing patients with diseases of known causation leads to the intuitive ordering of questions by likelihood of revealing significant findings. Thus, place of work or school, and place of recreation would be questions asked at the beginning of the interview. The common factor between the three cases was thus discovered without dredging their memories for implausible connections.

In conclusion it might be observed that at present, in the practice of infectious disease control, the framework of proven microbiological causes and modes of transmission enables statistical data to be interpreted confidently. Once outside of known causal pathways statistical associations are difficult to interpret and public health action usually is taken on the basis of clinical experience and instinct. Attention needs to be given to the mathematical description of this process.

REFERENCES

[1] Palmer, S. R., Jephcott, A. E., Rowland, A. J., Sylvester, D. G. H. (1981) Person to person spread of Salmonella typhimurium phage type 10 after a common source outbreak, Lancet i, 881-884

[2] Palmer, S. R., Caul, E. O. Donald, D. Kwantes, W., Tillett, H. (1985) An Outbreak of Shingles, Lancet, ii, 1108-1111.

[3] Peto, T. E. A., Gilks, C. F., Juel-Jenson, B. E. (1985) Clusters of Shingles, Lancet, ii, 1433.

[4] Palmer, S. R., Tillett, H., (1986) Shingles Clusters, Lancet, i, 273-274

[5] Morgan, G. J., Palmer, S. R., Onions, D., Anderson, M., Cartwright, R. A., Bentley, D. P. (1988) A cluster of three cases of aplastic anaemia in children, Clinical Laboratory Haematology, 10, 29-32

THE COMPUTATION OF GENERAL DETERMINISTIC AND STOCHASTIC EPIDEMICS

Gordon Reece

(Department of Engineering Mathematics University of Bristol)

ABSTRACT

This paper deals with the development of simple, robust and versatile time-dependent deterministic and stochastic models of epidemics suitable for implementation on a computer. Such models are needed if we are to make forecasts of the spread of HIV-1.

Section 2 describes the simplest (deterministic) models and goes on to show how these can easily be generalised to allow for different lengths of latency and infectivity periods. Section 3 deals with the direct simulation of a stochastic epidemic: Section 4 shows how to compute these directly.

Section 5 introduces a generalised "quasi-stochastic" model which can be computed directly and which retains some of the features of a fully stochastic approach. Section 6 shows how to develop a generalised deterministic model which is capable of predicting the behaviour of a disease as it spreads among groups which have different levels of susceptibility. Section 7 examines the results, which show similarity to the pattern of HIV-1, and explains how large secondary risk groups could succumb to such a disease long after it had run its course in the primary risk groups.

The results suggest, for example, that a health education program that is only 50% effective can cause a 90% fall in the number of cases over the succeeding eight years.

1 INTRODUCTION

1.1 Background

The advent of AIDS has provoked a great deal of unfounded speculation, much of it sensational, as to the future course of the disease. This has made more urgent the development of robust and flexible models capable of handling the more unusual aspects of the spread of HIV infection - the very long time-scales involved and the distinct mixing-rates of different risk groups and sub-groups. The present paper deals with the development of such models and goes on to show how they can be applied to the computational forecasting of the spread of HIV infection.

Let us make this point very clearly: the present paper is concerned with the epidemiological problem of modelling the spread of the Human Immunodeficiency Virus (HIV, now sadly renamed HIV-1 in the light of the appearance of a distinct but equally lethal form HIV-2). It is *not* concerned with the problem of forecasting the growth in the number of cases of AIDS. This latter problem remains for the present, at least, a statistical one, which is best treated by the methods of May & Anderson (1987) and of Anderson et al. (1987). In those papers, May, Anderson and their co-workers use sets of partial-differential equations to solve the problem of the spread of HIV-1 infection. In the present paper, a rather simpler, more transparent approach is developed. We shall establish methods which permit the direct prediction of the course of epidemics with very simple computer programs. It is the author's intention that these programs should be in the public domain.

With the models to be derived and applied in the present paper it would be possible to make forecasts based on the rate of spread of HIV infection that prevailed before the current increase in public awareness and the efforts being made to halt the spread. By comparing these forecasts with the actual figures it would be possible to assess the effectiveness of the current programmes of health education in terms of the reduction in the rate at which people continue to take risks.

1.2 Deterministic and stochastic models

Models used for the forecasting of epidemics fall into two categories: *deterministic* and *stochastic*. The difference between the two kinds of model is summarised in the difference between the two statements:

a. *Half the ten people in this room will catch cold this winter* (deterministic)

and

b. *Each of the ten people in this room has a fifty-fifty chance of catching cold this winter* (stochastic)

Using the statement (*b*) we can derive a great deal of information - not merely that half (on average) of the people will catch cold but that there is a 0.1% chance that none of the ten of us will catch cold, and so forth. Not surprisingly, since the stochastic approach gives us so much more information it is also a much more difficult and time-consuming method to use than the simple direct deterministic one. Because the deterministic approach glosses over much of the detail, it can sometimes lead to substantially different conclusions from those of a stochastic approach. In such cases, of course, the stochastic solution is the more informative one, if the original problem was actually a stochastic one (involving statements of chance or risk).

2 A DETERMINISTIC MODEL

In the simplest form of epidemic model, we have a population of initially *N susceptibles* and *a* initial *infectives,* where *a* and *N* are positive integers.

The deterministic problem is then

$$w = \frac{dC}{dt} = bCS \tag{1}$$

where *C* is the number of infectives, *S* the number of susceptibles and *b* the rate at which they mix, per unit time (*t*). Since *C*+*S*=*N*+*a*, we can write (1) as

$$\frac{dC}{dt} = bC(N + a - S) \tag{2}$$

We are (for convenience and just for the moment, while we look at this very simple case) assuming that every encounter between an infective and a susceptible results in the instantaneous transmission of infection.

Equation (2) can be integrated (Bailey, 1975):

$$C = a\frac{(N+a)}{N\exp\{-(N+a)bt\}+a}$$

i.e., differentiating with respect to *t*:

$$w = \frac{dC}{dt} = b\frac{aN(N+a)^2\exp\{(N+a)bt\}}{(N+a\exp\{(N+a)bt\})^2} \quad (3)$$

It is worth pointing out

(*a*) that Bailey's "*w*" is our "*w*/*b*": we are working with time *t*, whereas Bailey has transformed his time to *bt*

(*b*) that *b* is not non-dimensional

The role of the value of *b*, the mixing rate, is crucial. Total mixing of a population of $N+1$ people involves $N(N+1)/2$ encounters, so that a value of $b = 2/\{N(N+1)\}$ represents an average of one encounter per unit *t*. This is easily understood if we assume that the population is mixing at a uniform rate, such that an encounter can be expected in one unit of time (this may be 28.3 seconds or 16 weeks or 3.4 years,...). The chance of such an encounter being between an infective and a susceptible is equal to

$$\frac{\text{the number of pairings between a susceptible and an infective}}{\text{the total number of possible pairings}}$$

i.e.

$$\frac{CS}{N(N+1)/2}$$

or, in other words, $\dfrac{2CS}{N(N+1)}$

We shall work with the graph of *w* (new cases per unit time) against *t* (time). This is known as the *epidemic curve* and it is a much easier (and more sensitive) way of seeing what is happening than the curve we should get by plotting not the new cases per unit time at time *t* but the total number of cases (the sum, or integral, of the new cases up to time *t*).

Unfortunately, equation (2) assumes various things that are not in general true: that there is no period of *latency* (during which the victim is suffering from the disease, cannot catch it and cannot pass it on) and that once someone becomes infected he (or she - this will be assumed throughout) remains so for ever: i.e. we assume an infinitely-long period of *infectivity*. Once we abandon any of these assumptions, equation (2) no longer applies and we cannot expect to be able to solve the governing equation except numerically in general. We therefore show how to generalise (2) to allow for a variety of assumptions and how to solve the resulting equation numerically.

We introduce the notion of an *infectivity function* $f(t)$ which describes the behaviour of the disease in a given individual once he has been in contact with it. The simple assumption in (2) is shown in Figure 1: the value of f is zero before infection, becomes equal to 1 immediately upon contact with the disease and remains equal to 1 for ever after.

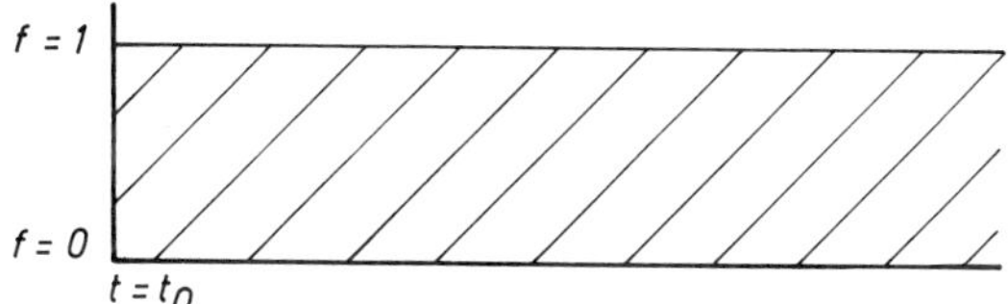

Figure 1 The infectivity function of a simple epidemic

Figure 2 shows a rather more general model: here there is a period of latency (E) after contact and the person remains infective for a finite time I after t=E, i.e. until t=E+I, whereupon the infectivity reverts to zero.

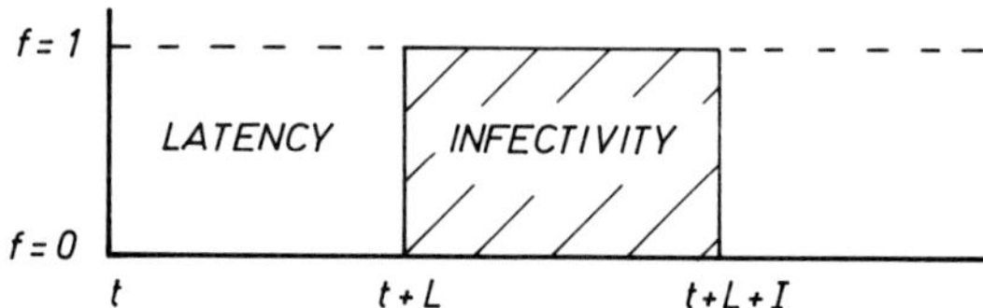

Figure 2 The infectivity function with latency and finite infectivity periods

Figure 3 shows a truly general form of *f* in which the infectivity varies between zero (totally unable to transmit the disease) and 1 (any contact between an infective and a susceptible passes on the disease).

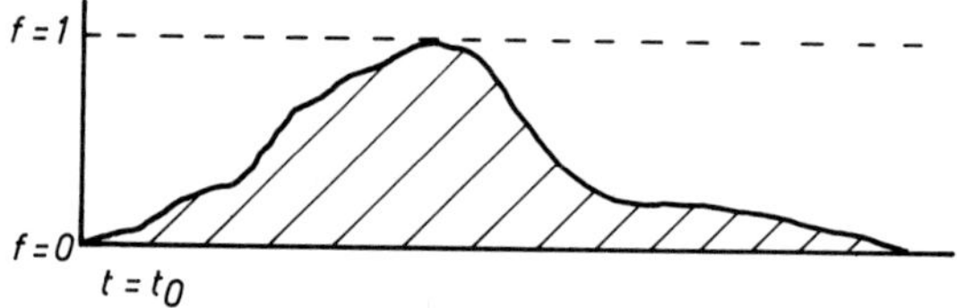

Figure 3 A completely general form of infectivity function

In Figures 1-3 the period of infectivity is shown shaded. Unless we indicate the contrary, it should be assumed that the state in which a person finds himself after t=E+I is that of a recovered immune: i.e. a "case" with susceptibility zero as well as zero infectivity. Once infected, a person is assumed permanently unable to catch the disease again. Of course, these assumptions can be modified by trivial adjustments to the program.

In the notation of Hethcote & Yorke (1984), the disease modelled here is of the form SEI: the progress of an individual member of the population is *Susceptible* (S), *Latent* or *Exposed* (E), *Infective* (I). There is no return to susceptibility nor is there any provision for *Removal* (R) of members of the population by death or isolation.

time	PROG1	eqn(3)
1	0.1818182	0.1818181
2	0.2109692	0.2133965
3	0.2432873	0.2485206
4	0.2785469	0.2868195
5	0.3162739	0.3275834
6	0.3556901	0.3697093
7	0.3956729	0.4116800
8	0.4347451	0.4516072
9	0.4711112	0.4873437
10	0.5027605	0.5166801
11	0.5276334	0.5376007
12	0.5438521	0.5485557
13	0.5499742	0.5486976
14	0.5452276	0.5380146
15	0.5296648	0.5173344
16	0.5041948	0.4881918
17	0.4704717	0.4525933
18	0.4306671	0.4127468
19	0.3871740	0.3708037
20	0.3423162	0.3286612
21	0.2981151	0.2878461
22	0.2561502	0.2494731
23	0.2175112	0.2142609
24	0.1828275	0.1825885
25	0.1523435	0.1545666
26	0.1260139	0.1301106
27	0.1035972	0.1090058

Table 1 The accuracy of the deterministic model: comparison of the analytical model with the output from the computer model.

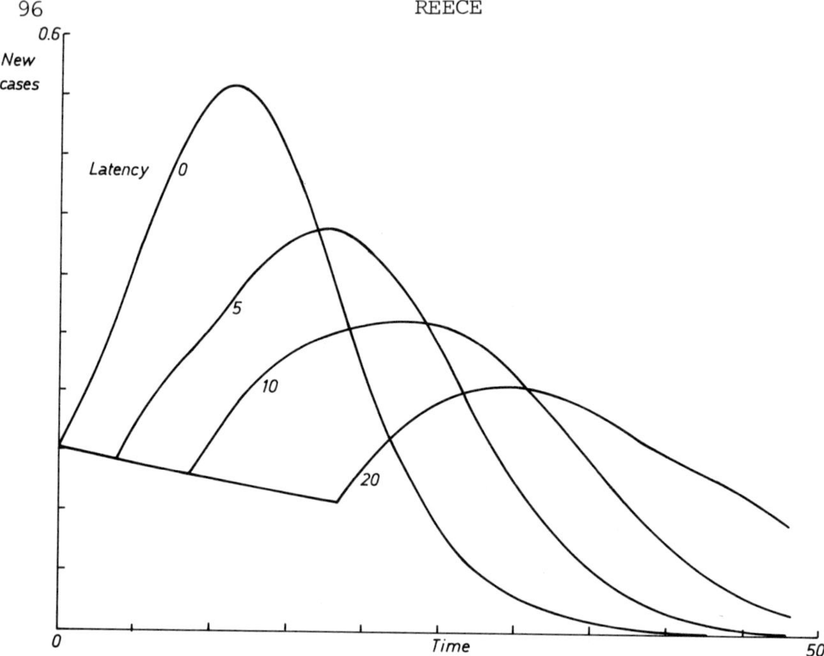

Figure 4 A deterministic epidemic with latency periods of 0, 5, 10, 20

The ordinate plotted is, in all the graphs, new cases appearing per unit time: this unit can be called "hours", "days" or what we like. For the moment, at least, we remember that we are taking the unit of time to be the time taken for one meeting to occur. So, if the rate of meeting of the population is one encounter per day, we take the day as the unit of time, and the number of new cases is calculated as the number of new cases per day. If the population mixes so that there is typically one encounter per 2.4 seconds, the unit of time will be 2.4 seconds and the epidemic curve will tell us how many new cases we should expect to see every 2.4 seconds. The minimum time for total mixing at a uniform rate is, of course, $N(N+1)/2$ units of time. Clearly, no more than one - and generally, on average, far less than one - infection can occur as the direct result of a single encounter.

We can use equation (4) to generate solutions of the problem for combinations of latency and infectivity. Finally, therefore, we show in Figure 6 the result of a deterministic forecast of the course of an epidemic among 1000 people. The disease has a latency period of 24 hours and an infectivity period of five days (120 hours).

Figure 7 shows the effect of having a latency period (10 days) greater than the period of infectivity (5 days) for N=10, together with the results for infectivity periods of 10 and 15 days. Clearly, the group of susceptibles infected during one burst of infectivity will not be able to pass on the infection until the burst is over, with the consequent possibility of waves of infection. This point is well illustrated by Figure 7.

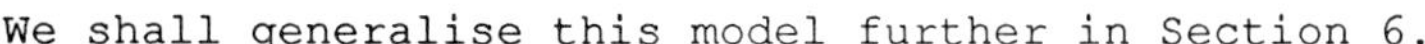
We shall generalise this model further in Section 6.

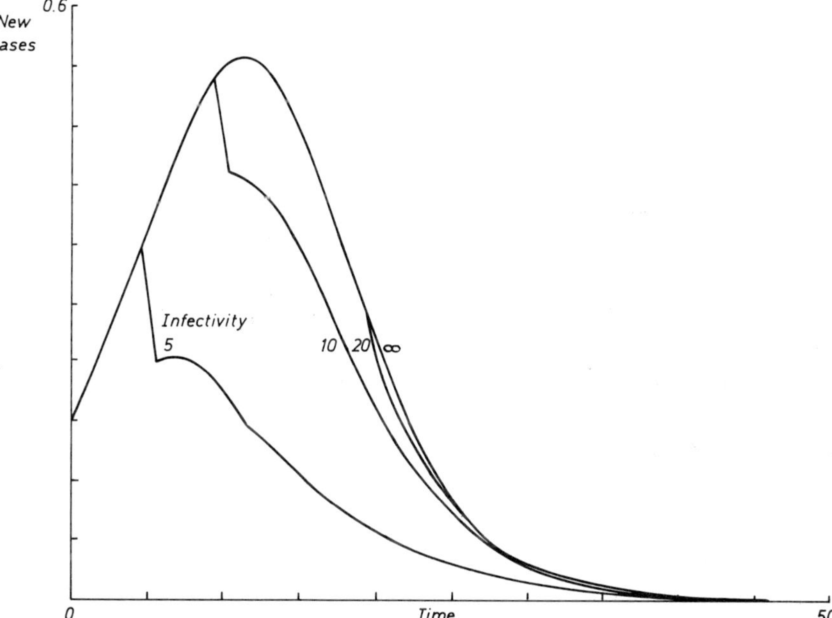

Figure 5 A deterministic epidemic with infectivity periods of 5, 10, 20 and infinity

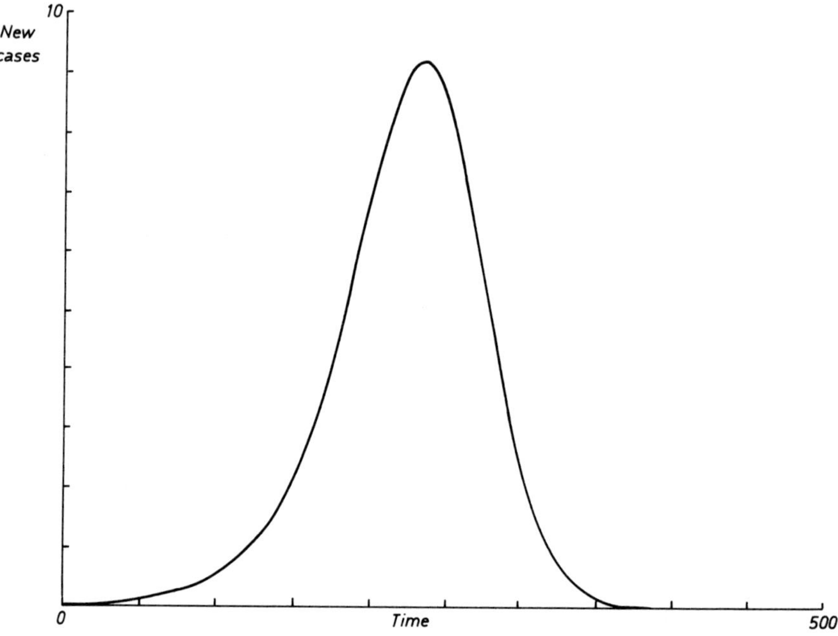

Figure 6 A deterministic epidemic among 1000 people, latency 24, infectivity 120

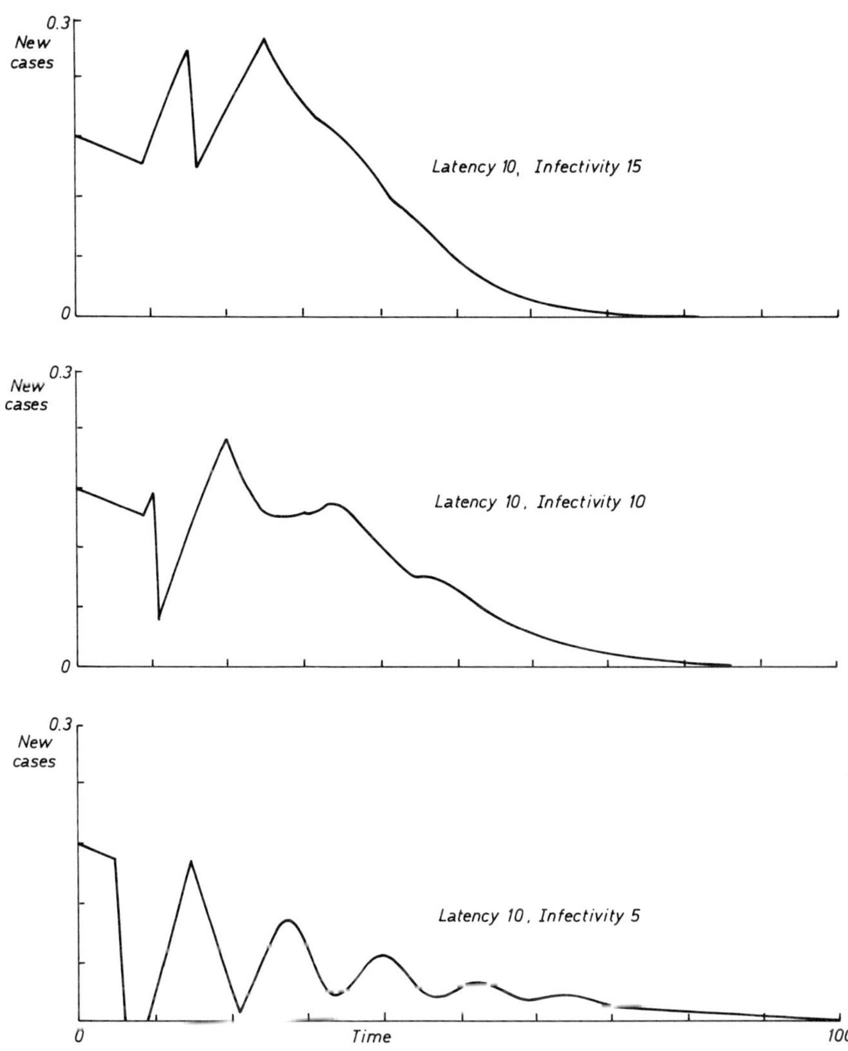

Figure 7 A deterministic epidemic among 10 people with latency 10, infectivity 5, 10, 15

3 STOCHASTIC MODELLING

Various attempts have been made in the past to produce a stochastic model of epidemics which was capable of generalisation to non-trivial problems. By non-trivial we mean problems involving large populations, non-zero latency periods and finite periods of infectivity. None of these attempts appears to have led to a satisfactory practicable solution of the problem.

One method which was regarded as impossibly extravagant in computer time until recently (see, e.g., Frauenthal, 1980) is no longer out of the question: we can use a computer to *simulate* an epidemic using the computer effectively as a many-sided die, which we roll millions of times. Kramer & Reynolds (1981) published the results of such a simulation. Sadly, Kramer & Reynolds failed to provide even details of how many runs they performed, so that there is no way of assessing the accuracy of their simulation procedures from the information they published. We shall be particularly concerned to establish the reliability of the simulation process, so that we can use the results as the basis for determining the accuracy of our procedures for simulation. There is little point in indulging in the expense of a stochastic simulation unless we can be sure of its accuracy.

We approach the problem as follows. We consider, as in the deterministic case, the effect of introducing (say) one infective into a population of N susceptibles. We again take the unit of time as that during which one encounter will occur. This has the advantage that we need not waste time picking multiple random pairs from a finite population: such processes are notoriously slow especially if we have to avoid "replacement", i.e. the danger of picking the same person twice.

A pair of members of the population is picked at random. If and only if it consists of an infective and a susceptible does it lead to a new infection. We shall assume for the moment an f of the type in Figure 1, a simple epidemic. Let us call the unit of time a "day". We repeat the process for the next "day", and so forth for a reasonable number of "days". If the population N=10 (+1) it takes about 50 "days" for the epidemic to run its course. For N=20 it takes about 80 days. We then repeat the whole process from day zero, do this 10000 times and then average the number of new infections per day. Clearly, as there is just one pairing per day, there can be either one infection or no infections each day for each simulated epidemic. The resulting graphs for simple epidemics of N=10 and N=20 are shown in Figures 8 and 9. These were generated using the program EP2.

The discrepancy between the curves and the exact solutions, taken from Mansfield & Hensley (1960), and shown on Figures 8 and 9, is due not to the inaccuracy of the simulation but to the fact that we have stipulated a fixed time interval between events: the actual intervals would be random, with a mean as in our case, but spread about that mean. The error is less than 5%. We have shown in each case the deterministic solution for the same problem and it is clear that the effect of using a fixed time interval is to make the solutions "more deterministic" than the true stochastic solution. The maximum in all cases is at roughly the same point. The method we have used is perhaps best described as "quasi-stochastic".

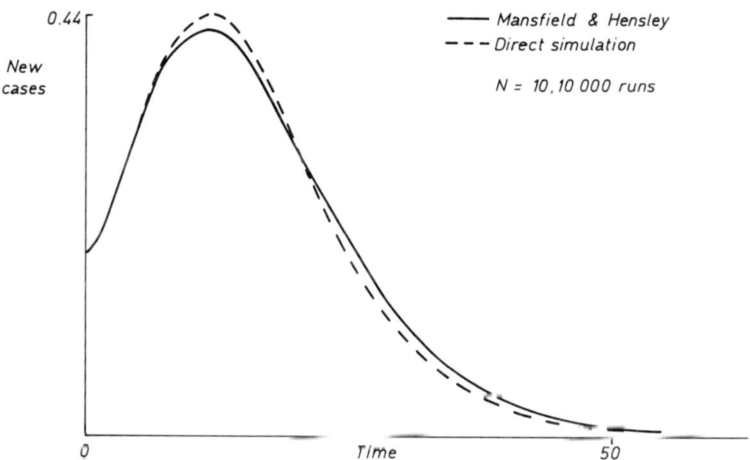

Figure 8 Direct simulation of a stochastic epidemic, N=10

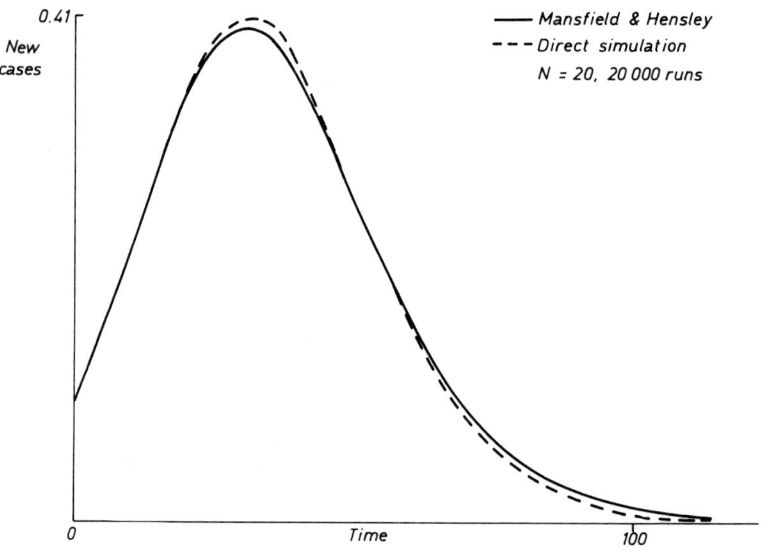

Figure 9 Direct simulation of a stochastic epidemic, N=20

If we retain the information in all cases as to when each member of the population was first infected with the disease, we can easily generalise the method to allow for infectivity functions *f* of the types shown in Figures 2 and 3. Using an *f* as in Figure 2, with latency periods of 5 and 10 "days", we get the graphs shown in Figure 9 for a population of 10. Figures 8-10 are taken from Hill (1986): in Hill (1986) there are further examples of the application of the method for various periods of latency and infectivity and for populations of 10 and 20.

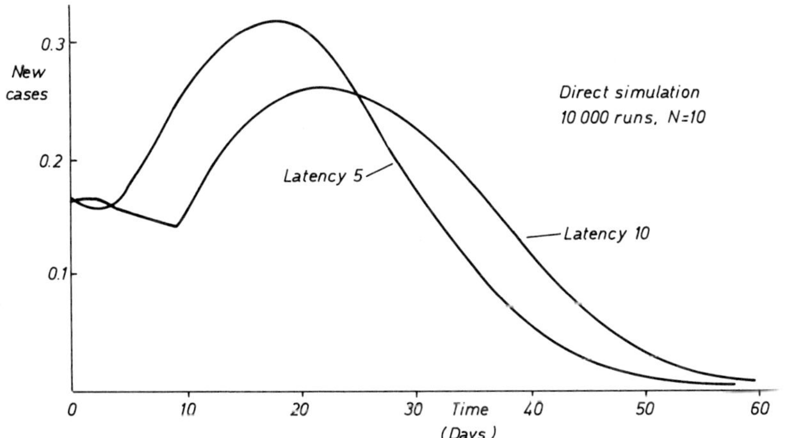

Figure 10 Direct simulation of a stochastic epidemic, N=10, latency 5,10

4 DIRECT CALCULATION OF SIMPLE STOCHASTIC EPIDEMICS

If, yet again, we consider the effect of a single encounter, it will lead to either one new case or no new cases. If we have r cases on "day" t, these will arise either

* if on day t-1 there were r cases and there are no new cases on day t-1 or

* if on day t-1 there were r-1 cases and there is one new case on day t-1

As these possibilities are mutually exclusive, the probability $P(r,t)$ of having exactly r cases on day t will be given by their sum

$$P(r,t) = P(r-1,t-1).b(r-1)(N+2-r) + P(r,t-1)\{1 - br(N+1-r)\} \quad (5)$$

This expression tells us the probability that there will be exactly r cases on day t provided that we know the probabilities on the previous day. But we know that $P(1,0)=1$, as we start with exactly one infective at time t=0.

We have chosen to take as our starting point the introduction of exactly one initial infective into a healthy population: it is a trivial extension of the analysis to set the initial condition to cover the case of $a>1$ initial infectives. Here, for example, we should simply have to set $P(a,0)=1$. Appropriate provision has been made in the computer program.

The probabilities $P(r,1)$ $(r=0,1)$; $P(r,2)$ $(r=0,1,2)$... can be generated. Clearly no more than $r+1$ cases can be generated by r pairings. We can determine the mean of the total number of cases at time t simply by calculating

$$\sum_{r=1}^{N+1} rP(r,t)$$

For the simple epidemic the $P(r,t)$ must sum to 1.0 on any given "day" - a statement of the fact that all epidemics must pass through t with just one value of r.

We therefore have only to calculate the values of $P(r,t)$ and of the moment of $P(r,t)$ about $r=0$ at each time t. We require knowledge at this stage only of $P(r,t)$ and of $P(r,t-1)$ together with $P(r-1,t-1)$. So we need retain just two vectors of (maximum) length N at any time. When $P(r,t+1)$ is being calculated, $P(r,t-1)$ can be discarded for all r.

To obtain the epidemic curve, we must subtract the stochastic mean $m(t-1)$ at time $t-1$ from the value $m(t)$ at time t. The resulting forecasts for $N=10$ and $N=20$ are shown in Figures 11 and 12. The results of the direct simulations of Section 2 are shown and they are very close indeed.

If we now consider the discrepancy between the analytic solutions and the present ones, we can see that since the analytic ones assume a continuous path through time and we have chosen to take uniform time steps, we should be able to generate the analytical solutions simply by reducing the time step: i.e. by reducing the value of b. That this is indeed the case is clear from Figure 13, in which we show the results of reducing the value of b from its current setting

$$b_0 = 2/\{N(N+1)\}$$

to 0.1 b_0 and then to 0.01 b_0 for $N=10$: the exact solution (Bailey, 1975) is also displayed. It is clear that the process converges (numerically) to the continuous case. We have therefore a limiting process which can calculate *directly* the values of the mean of any simple stochastic epidemic.

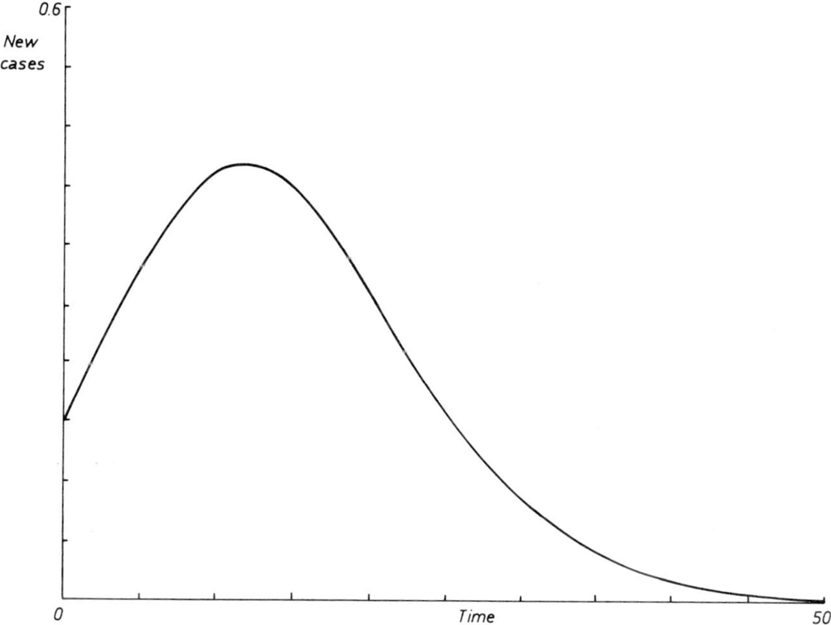

Figure 11 Direct calculation of a simple stochastic epidemic, N=10

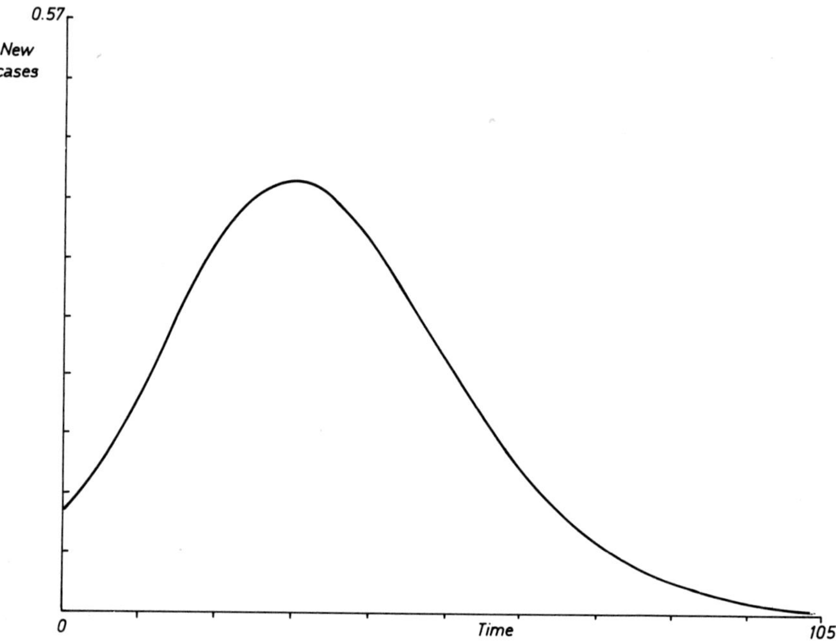

Figure 12 Direct calculation of a simple stochastic epidemic, N=20

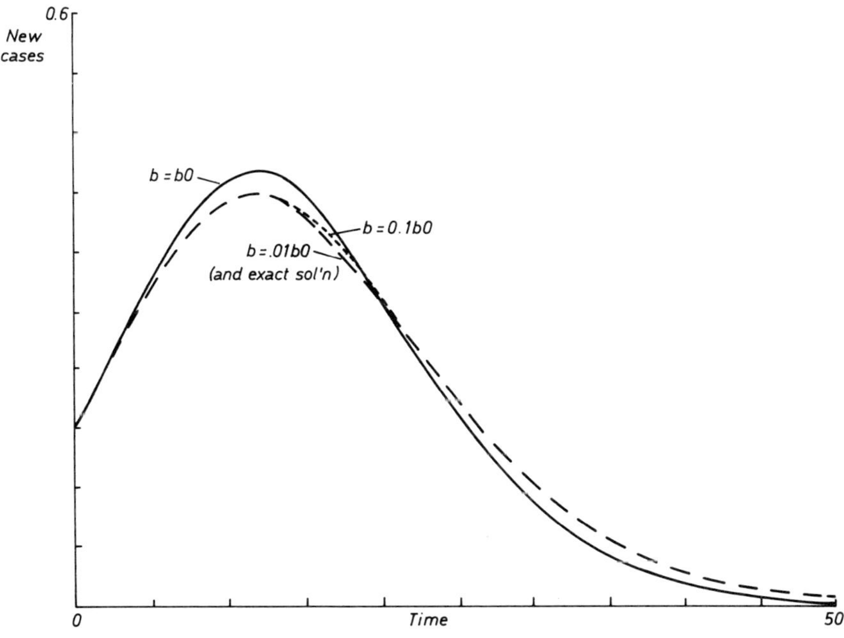

Figure 13 Comparison of exact and directly-calculated solutions of a stochastic epidemic, N=10

We can, of course, also derive the probability distribution of a simple stochastic epidemic, using the same technique, this time without taking moments.

Since the memory requirements of our procedure are dictated by the need to carry forward two vectors of length N, we can calculate the stochastic mean course of epidemics involving up to $M/N/2$ people if M is the number of numbers we can store on our computer after making room for the fixed overheads of the scheme (the program and the parameters).

We show the result of calculating a simple stochastic epidemic of 100 people. Special devices have to be adopted to get round the problem of adding together a very large number of very large numbers, which is what is required by our formula. The graphs shown were generated using the program EP3 with N=100, b=b_0.

By plotting

$$z = w/\{b(N+1)^2\}$$

against (6)

$$t' = (N+1)bt - \log N$$

following Williams (1965) we can confirm that our model of a simple stochastic epidemic gives Williams' result that there is a single stochastic epidemic curve which is rapidly approached as the population grows. This result is shown in Figure 14 for a population of 100. The theoretical curve (Williams, 1965) is indistinguishable from the one shown.

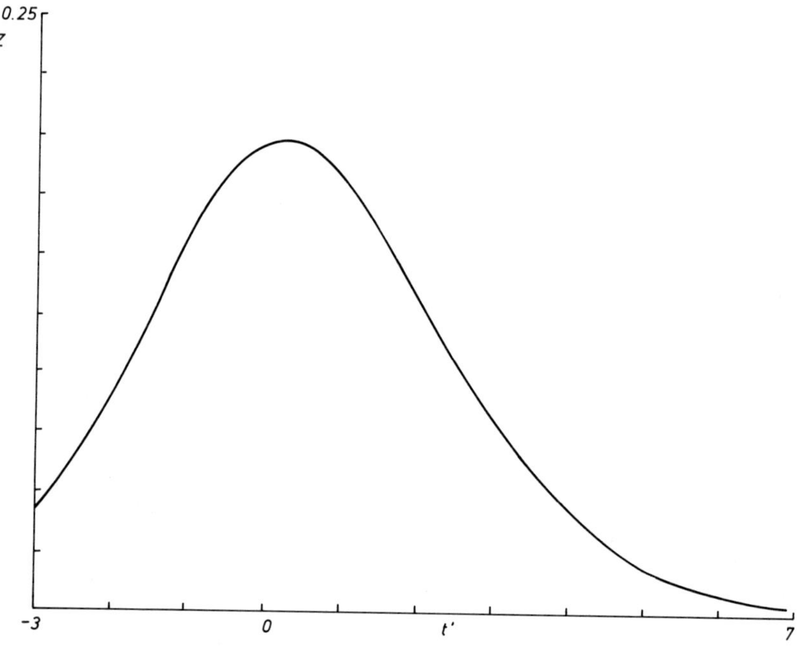

Figure 14 Direct calculation of a simple stochastic epidemic, N=100, using the transformations (6)

5 A QUASI-STOCHASTIC MODEL OF GENERAL EPIDEMICS

We can generalise the approach of Section 3 as follows. If on "day" t there are r infectives including one who caught the disease on day $i<t$, this will follow as before from either r-1 infectives on day t-1 including one dating from i, together with a new infection on day t-1, or from r cases at t-1 including one dating from i and no new infection. If an infectivity function f is introduced, we shall need to know the history

(date of infection) of each infective on any day t. This will tell us the infectivity of the r or r-1 cases present on day t-1.

A truly stochastic approach would allow for the fact that the infectivity of the r or r-1 cases on any given day is itself a stochastic variable. We should need to store an unacceptably large amount of information, in principle going back to day 0, in order to keep track of the probabilities. We compromise as follows: on each day we take the infectivity of r cases including one generated on day i as being the mean infectivity rather than the actual infectivity with its dispersion about the mean. Inevitably this approach will tend to make the progress of the epidemic more deterministic than it should be in principle. We shall show that the discrepancies between our approach and the results obtained from the direct simulation approach of Section 2 are not unacceptable, and they give us a better feel for the quality of our forecasts than we should derive from a purely deterministic approach.

The formula we use is the following one:

$$P(r,t,i) = P(r-1,t-1,i)br_1(N+2-r) + P(r,t-1,i)\{1-br_2(N+1-r)\} \qquad (7)$$

where r_1 is the mean infectivity of r-1 cases on day t-1, r_2 is the mean infectivity of r cases on day t-1

$$r_2 = r\frac{\left\{\sum_{k=1}^{t-2} f(t-k)P(r,t,k)\right\}}{\sum_{k=1}^{t-2}\{P(r,t,k)\}} \qquad (8)$$

and r_1 can be derived from this formula simply by replacing r by r-1 everywhere.

Using EP4 to implement our formula, we can calculate the quasi-stochastic mean corresponding to the result of the same problem solved using the direct simulation approach of Section 2.

We show in Figures 15 and 16 the results corresponding to those of Figures 4 and 5. We see that the curves err slightly on the "deterministic" side of those in Figure 10, which, as we must assume in the light of Figure 13, themselves err slightly in the same direction.

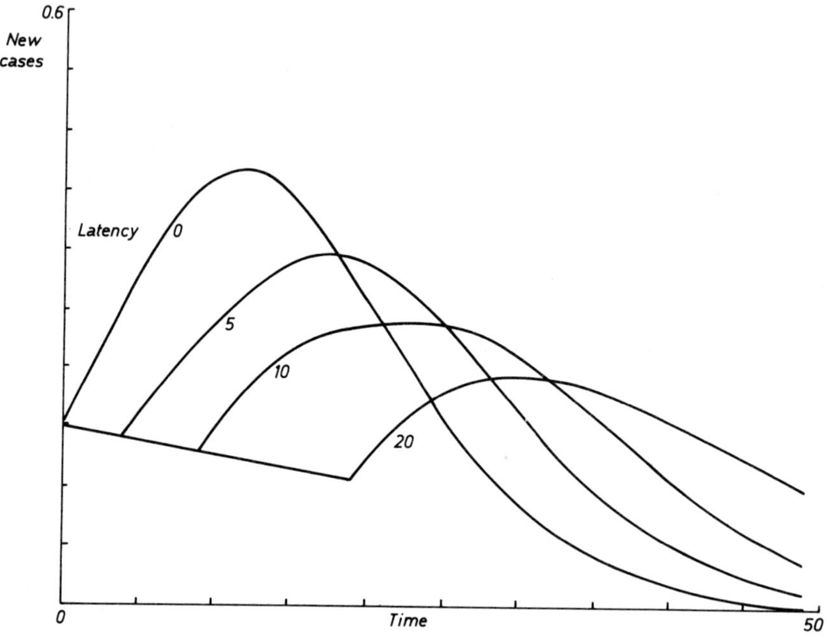

Figure 15 A stochastic epidemic with latency periods of 0, 5, 10, 20

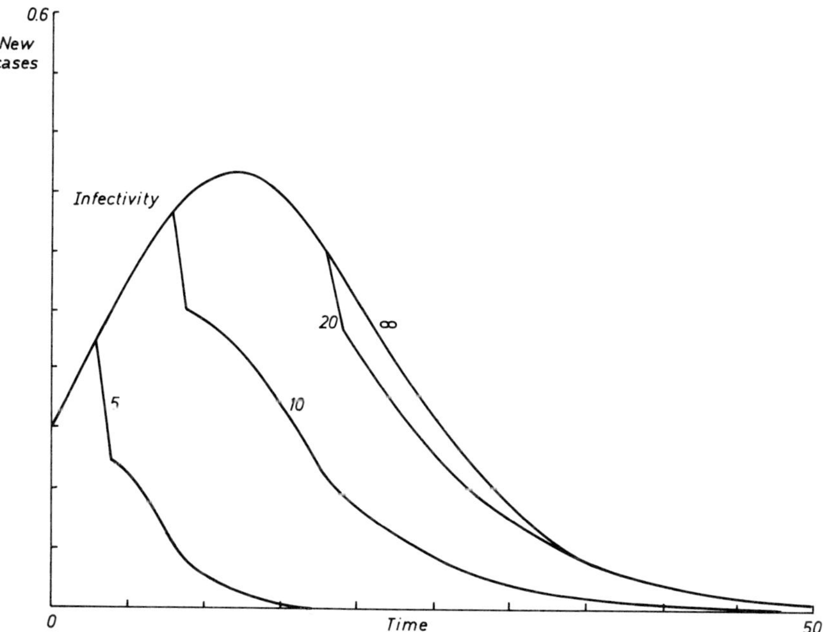

Figure 16 A stochastic epidemic with infectivity periods of 5, 10, 20, infinity

Figure 17 illustrates the case where we have a latency period of 10 days and infectivity periods of 5, 10 and 15 days, i.e. corresponding to Figure 7. We see how much more fragile the stochastic epidemic is than its deterministic counterpart: just as the actual values of the deterministic solutions are higher than those of the stochastic version, equally Figure 17 shows that a stochastic epidemic is less likely to resume its course after plunging to zero than is the curve we get (Figure 7) of the much sturdier deterministic solution. We are thus entitled to use deterministic solutions as a kind of "worst case" bound for the mean.

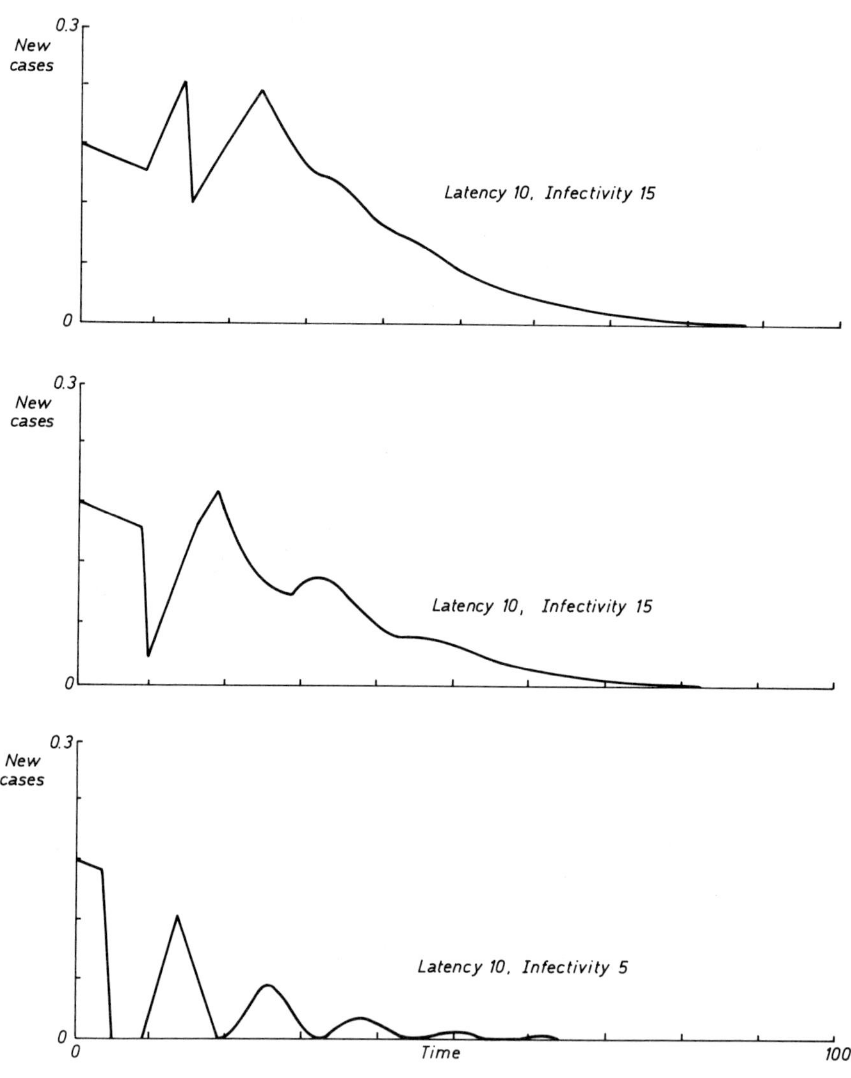

Figure 17 A stochastic epidemic with latency 10, infectivity 5, 10, 15

We show in Figure 18 the result of quasi-stochastic forecasts of epidemics involving 60 people suffering from diseases with latency periods of 0 and 10 weeks and an infectivity period of 350 weeks, with a mixing rate of b_0 - i.e. one encounter per week.

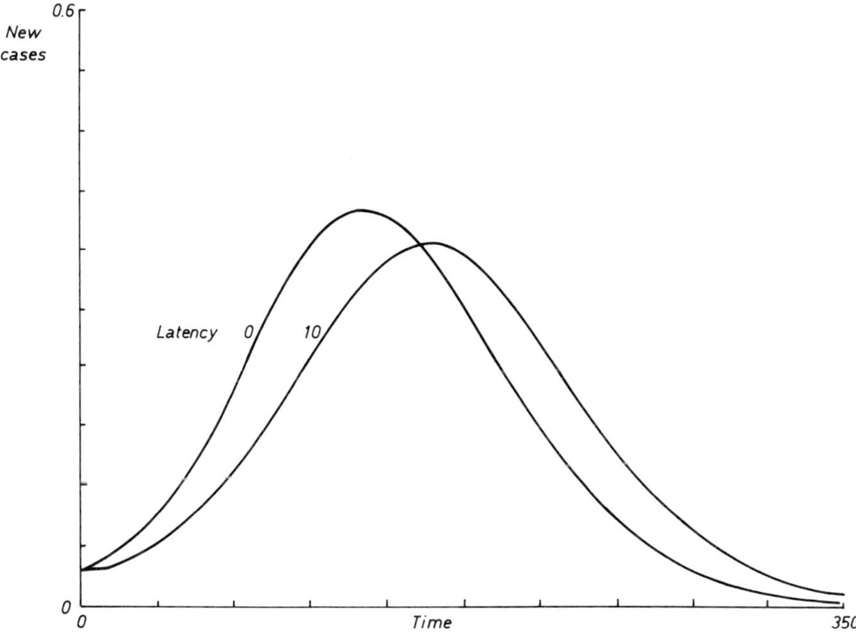

Figure 18 A stochastic epidemic for N=60, with latency 0, 10 and infinitely-long infectivity

6 A DETERMINISTIC MULTI-GROUP MODEL

All epidemics are deterministic at the outset. By asserting that we can inject exactly one infective into a healthy population at precisely time $t=0$ we are making a deterministic statement. It is only with the passage of time that any of our models allows uncertainty to enter our calculations. The extent to which this will occur will be directly related to the extent to which we have predetermined the outcome of the epidemic by the imposition of our initial conditions.

Williams, for example, showed (Williams, 1965) that the outcome of an epidemic among 20 people was virtually determined if we assumed 4 initial infectives rather than one. In practice, we rarely become aware of the progress or seriousness of an epidemic until it has affected a considerable number of people. In the case of the particular epidemic which initially excited our attention - the "AIDS virus" - has already spread to 30 000 people in the United Kingdom (January 1987, U.K. Department of Health & Social Security). We shall examine the extent to which in a population greater than 20, the situation at time t=0 determines the outcome of the epidemic. Figure 19 shows the forecasts of a simple stochastic epidemic in a population of 60 with a number of initial infectives varying from 1 to 20. These results are further compared in Figure 20 with the deterministic model for a population of 60 with the corresponding number of initial infectives. It is strikingly clear that if 20 out of 60 already have the disease the stochastic mean forecast is effectively identical to that given by the deterministic model.

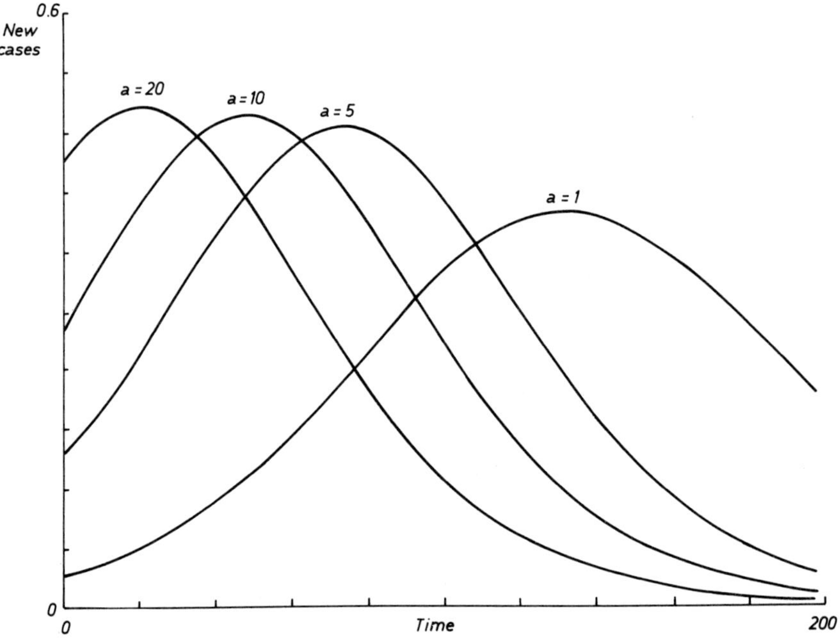

Figure 19 A stochastic epidemic with N=60, for 1, 5, 10, 20 initial infectives

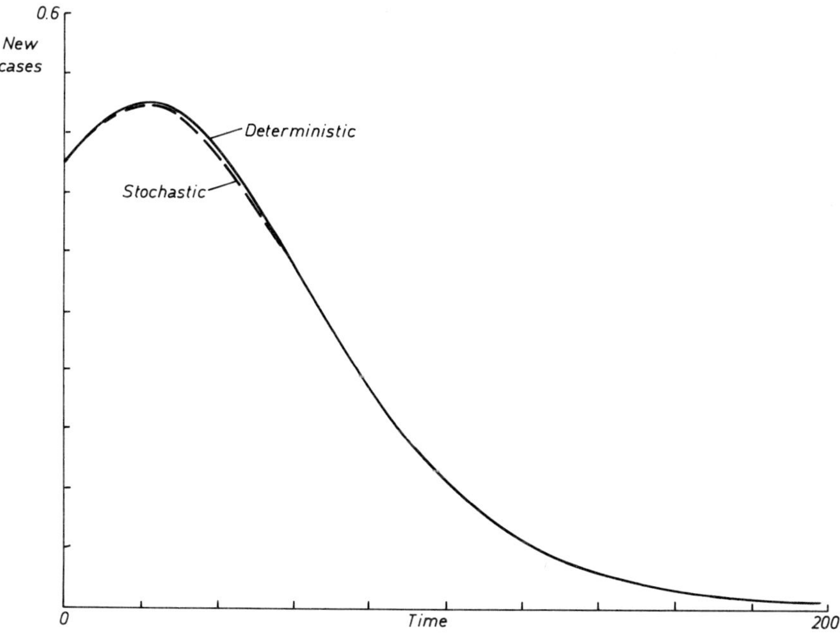

Figure 20 Comparison of deterministic and stochastic models for N=60, with 20 initial infectives

We note that

* a truly stochastic model of a general epidemic would be very expensive to use, requiring more computational power than is currently available;

* in practice we are normally faced with the problem of forecasting the further progress of a disease which has already taken hold to such an extent that much of the indeterminacy has already been eliminated at the (effective) outset;

* the number of people who have to have the disease before the further course can be satisfactorily forecast using a deterministic model is not great: using Williams' result (Figure 14 above) and the information in Figures 19 and 20 we can see that this number is not greater than 20%. The current rate of HIV-1 infection in high-risk groups in high-risk areas is over 30%.

We therefore consider the problem of devising a satisfactory general epidemic model for interacting populations (or groups within a population). The distinguishing characteristic of a group is its rate of mixing both within itself and in its interaction with other groups. The mixing rate includes the rate at which the disease spreads as a result of the particular type of mixing between groups.

The number of new cases per unit time for a simple deterministic epidemic is:

$$\frac{dC_i}{dt} = \left\{\sum_j b_{ji} C_j\right\} (N_i - C_i) \tag{9}$$

and this approach can be generalised exactly as in equation (4) above to allow for an infectivity function f:

$$w_i(t) = \left\{\sum_j b_{ji}\left(\int_0^t f(t-x) w_j(x) dx\right)\right\}\left\{N_i - \int_0^t w_i(x) dx\right\} \tag{10}$$

We now have a transmission matrix $b(j,i)$, the elements of which are the rates at which group j can be expected to transmit the disease to group i. The transmission rates are assumed normalised to the value of b_0

$$b_0 = 2/\{N(N-1)\}$$

corresponding to the fraction of total mixing represented by one pairing in a population of N, where N is the total population summed over all the groups. We are now obliged to break with the convention of starting with N susceptibles and a infectives as our infectives can, of course, be introduced into any of the groups: there is no *a priori* home for them.

The model is effectively the same as that used by Hethcote, Yorke & Nold (1982) to calculate the steady-state ("endemic") solutions of the equations (9). A computer program for this purpose is listed in Hethcote & Yorke (1984). A similar approach has been used by Knox (1986) to find steady-state solutions for a model of the HIV-1 problem. We shall be concerned with the control of an epidemic when it is at the early stages, long before it is clear whether there is an endemic solution - i.e. before we know whether the population can survive with the disease rumbling along and maybe erupting from time to time, as is the case, by definition, for all diseases that do not either disappear or threaten to extinguish their hosts. We shall therefore be concerned to derive time-dependent solutions. The incorporation of the infectivity function, with provision for non-zero latency period and finite duration of infectivity, is essential. Time-dependent solutions for equations (9) were obtained for a two-group model by Kemper (1980), but they lacked provision for latency and infectivity.

Some care is required in calculating the values of $b(j,i)$ from any given set of data: the value of $b(j,i)$ has to be chosen to represent the observed transmission rate from group j to group i (not necessarily, of course, the same as that from group i to group j) as a fraction of the rate at which the disease would have been expected to spread as a result of pairings at a rate b_0.

7 MODELLING AIDS - CONCLUSIONS

A reasonable guess at the form of the infectivity function f for HIV-1 can be made on the basis of current research. It would appear that the virus becomes transmissible within about 20 days of first infection, with a peak of infectivity at around the time of sero-conversion (about 60 days after infection) and a decay of infectivity following the advent of symptoms (Weber et al., 1987).

Using EP5 to implement the generalised multi-group deterministic model developed in Section 7, we obtain the results shown in Figure 21 for a disease involving two groups. The disease has a latency period of three weeks and an infectivity period of 150 weeks. The one group comprises 6% of the total population and it is this group in which the infective appears at time t=0. The mixing-rates have been chosen to illustrate the fact that an epidemic can sweep inexorably through one part of a population and then, seemingly unconnected with the earlier epidemic, but equally inexorably, a similar epidemic of the same disease is seen to sweep through the rest of the population. For the spread of the disease, the matrix of $b(j,i)$ is assumed to be

$$\begin{pmatrix} 1000b_0 & b_0 \\ b_0 & 10b_0 \end{pmatrix} \tag{11}$$

where b_0=2/1000/1001, i.e. about .000002. This means that we have assumed that members of group 1 transmit the disease 1000 times as fast among themselves as they do to members of group 2: the disease spreads ten times as fast among members of group 2 as it does from group 1 to group 2 (and vice-versa).

This model can easily be used to simulate spatial spread of a deterministic epidemic, since the $b(j,i)$ can be the observed rate of transmission as between two groups that are physically separated.

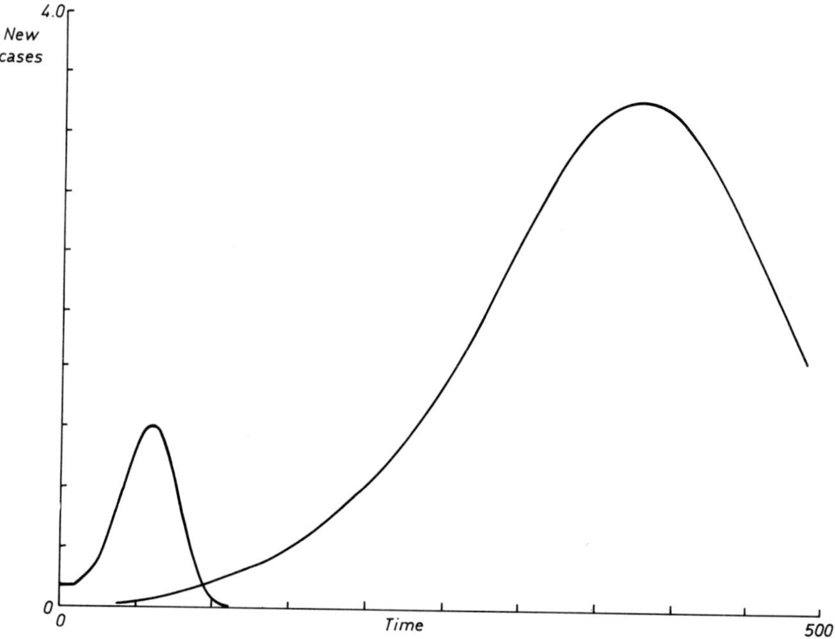

Figure 21 A deterministic epidemic among a population with two well-defined subgroups (N_1=60 and N_2=940)

Finally, it will be noted that we are assuming throughout the models described that an infective remains available for pairing for all time. This is to assume effectively that there are no withdrawals from the population: in the case of HIV-1, for example, there have been (UK, end of 1986) about 300 withdrawals by death from a population of (say) 20 million people at risk, of whom 30 000 are already infected. Withdrawals therefore need not concern us at this stage, at least. Any other kind of withdrawal, such as the result of the modification induced by health education of the behaviour of the population at risk, is better modelled by means of a modified value of mixing rate (since the people will continue to mix but - we trust - will spread the disease less rapidly as a result of their modified behaviour) rather than by tampering with the overall size of the population involved.

In Figure 22, we show the result of a similar calculation to that in Figure 21: this time with a mixing rate among the 94% group among themselves - i.e. $b(2,2)$ - which is reduced to 50% of its former value after 100 weeks. This graph illustrates both the power of the model and that of health education. In Figure 23 we see the effect of a health-education programme introduced after 50 weeks. The similarity between Figures 22 and 23 suggests that it is largely the mixing-rate $b(2,2)$ among the larger group that is influential in determining the course of the epidemic among that group even at that early stage, rather than the other $b(i,j)$, even though most of the infectives at that stage still belong to the smaller group.

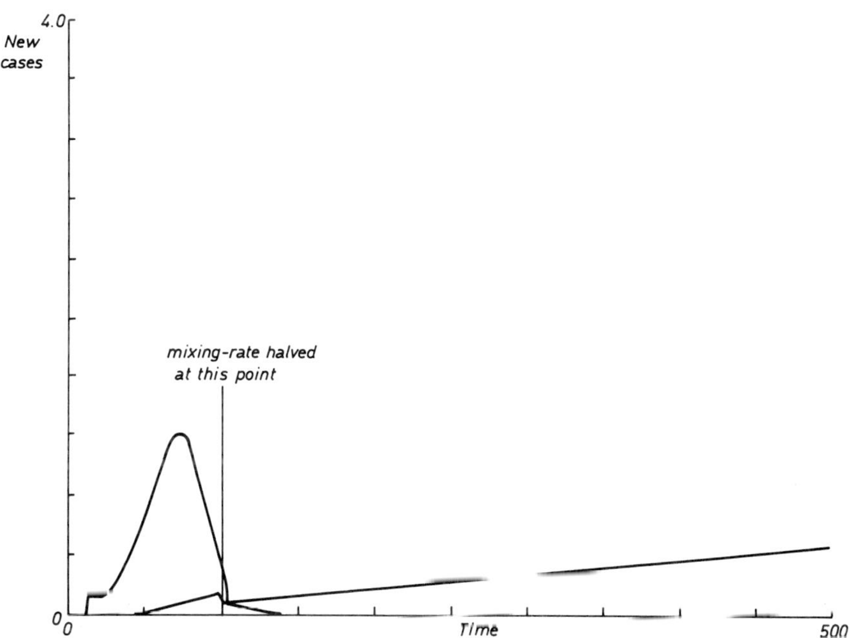

Figure 22 As Figure 21, but showing the effect of health education

The striking conclusion from the graphs in Figures 21 and 22 is that even if it is only 50% successful a health-education programme can reduce the number of cases of disease like HIV-1 by 90% over a period of 10 years. By 50% successful we mean that the rate of mixing, i.e. of risk-taking, is reduced to half of its previous value. From Figures 22 and 23 we can see that this result holds even if the intervention occurs at what would seem to be quite a late stage in the evolution of the disease among a small subgroup within which the original infection is supposed to have occurred.

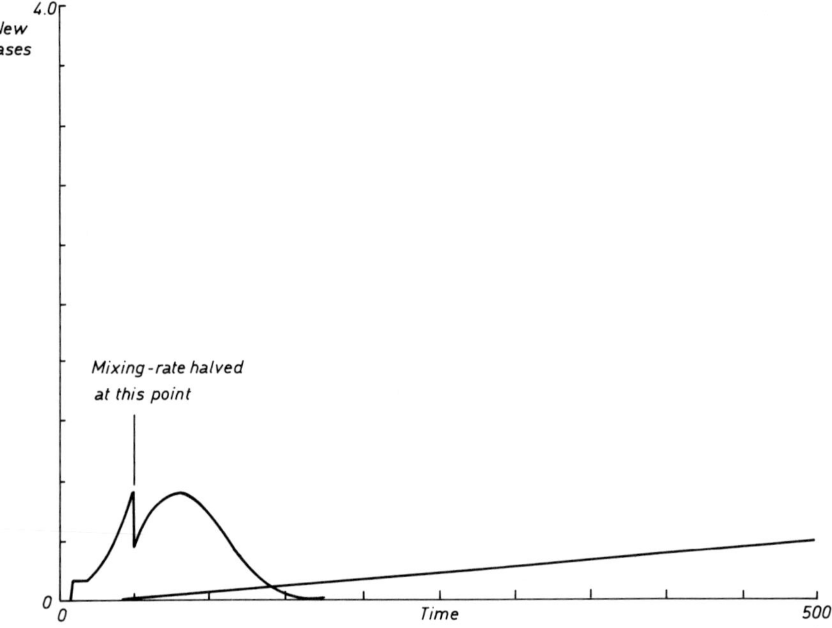

Figure 23 As Figure 22, but with earlier intervention

Our crude attempt at modelling the spread of HIV-1 through a small community could so easily be refined if we had access to reasonable data concerning the lifestyles of various groups within the general population. In our computer program EP5 we have provided (arbitrarily) for the division of any population into ten subgroups: in the case of HIV-1 these would be such groups as homosexual men (stratified by, e.g., age), bisexual men, predominantly-heterosexual men, heterosexual women, intravenous drug-users and so forth. If only we had better data, such as that being accumulated by Coxon (1986) and McManus & McEvoy (1987), we could now make forecasts of how the disease would spread in the absence of any modification of lifestyles, how it will spread in the light of known changes in people's behaviour and how it would spread if we could target particular risk-groups and convince them that they should modify their behaviour in the interest of the community at large.

The most important result that can be derived from the work of Hill (1986) is the (negative) conclusion that there was no necessary foundation for the widespread conjecture that a mechanism must exist to increase the susceptibility to HIV-1 of the population at risk somehow in line with the rate at which they took risks. This was an unwarranted conclusion drawn from the fact that there *seemed* to be a disproportionately large presence of very-high-risk people in the first batch of victims of the disease. There are two points to be made:

* we do not know what constitutes either "disproportionately" or "very-high-risk", simply because (in the absence of accurate up-to-date information about gay and IV-drug-users' lifestyles) we do not know what the "norm" is, let alone the distribution of the rate of risk-taking about that "norm"

* because the process is not a simple linear one, the people running particularly high risks will necessarily be represented more than proportionately among the early cases.

Hill (1986) showed what is after all only common sense: that the high-risk population succumbs at an early stage in the epidemic, leaving few (or no) high-risk members of the population to succumb in the later stages. There will therefore in the last stages of the epidemic be a preponderance of low-risk people: conversely, there will have to be a disproportionately large number of high-risk people in the early stages. (*The law of conservation of people.*) This is obvious. What is not obvious is the ratios involved: these will depend on the distribution of lifestyles (rate of risktaking). As no-one yet has such information it is simply impossible to draw any conclusions merely on the basis that the initial victims include a particular fraction of very-high-risk people, however high that fraction might *seem* to be.

Similar conclusions to those of Hill (1986) have since been drawn by Peto (1986) on the basis of what appears to be a deterministic approach.

There is thus no need to look for reasons (such as rectal "trauma", lesions, etc.) why high-risk people should become ultra-susceptible. There is no evidence that they do. However, the search for such explanations has led in turn to an inordinate preoccupation with the possibility of accidental transmission through lesions anywhere on the body - in the absence of a significant number of cases of HIV-1 infection requiring any such explanation.

In one sense this is reassuring to the epidemiologist studying HIV-1: there need be no magical "missing ingredient" to explain the known facts. In another sense, this is very worrying, as it means that anyone is at risk at any time - even the first time they run risks, just as much as the hundredth time.

According to Tovey (1987), Peto (1986) asserts that the risk of infection from a single act of penetrative intercourse with an HIV-1-seropositive partner is about 1%. This is *not* the case: Peto merely announced the consequence of *postulating* such a degree of infectivity. We simply do not have enough information to make such a definite assertion. The information should be available from the work of Coxon (1986) when that is completed. McManus and McEvoy (1987) have shown that the work is likely to be successful. They have not, unlike Coxon, investigated frequencies of risk-taking, so that we still lack objective information to determine appropriate values of b for the population: we do not yet have even a mean value, though, as we have seen, this would not necessarily be particularly helpful in the light of Hill's results (Hill, 1986). It is vital to bear in mind the fact that it is only encounters that involve a risk of the transmission of the disease that need concern us. A mere change of partners - and certainly a mere casual encounter - does not necessarily involve any risk of transmission of the disease. It is thus not possible to derive useful information even from a crude rate-of-change-of-partners figure: what we need is (at the very least) a mean rate-of-change of risk-partner. When seeking this information it is necessary to keep a chronological diary of risk-taking: for example, if A and B are otherwise strictly-monogamous partners until A meets C, B may then become a risk-partner of A although he may never have had contact with anyone other than A. Because, as we have seen from Hill's work, the variation in degree of risk-taking is crucial to any serious model, a simple mean figure is almost certainly not sufficient. This point has eluded even such meticulous researchers as May & Anderson (1987): see Reece (1987). It would appear that we must await the outcome of Coxon's work (see, e.g., Coxon, 1986) for even a glimmer of the answer.

8 REFERENCES

Anderson, R.M., Medley, G.F., Blythe, S.P., Johnson, A.M., "Is it possible to predict the minimum size of the acquired immunodeficiency syndrome (AIDS) epidemic in the United Kingdom?", *Lancet*, 1987 (i), pp 1073-1075.

Bailey, N.T.J. *The Mathematical Theory of Infectious Diseases*, Griffin, London, 1975 (2nd Edition).

Cooke, K.L. and Yorke, J.A. "Some equations modelling growth processes and gonorrhea epidemics", *Math. Biosci.*, 16, pp 75-101, 1973.

Coxon, A.P.M., *Report of Pilot Study: Project on Sexual Lifestyles of Non-Heterosexual Males*, Sociological Research Unit, University College, Cardiff, 1986.

Frauenthal, J.C. *Mathematical Modelling in Epidemiology*, Springer, New York, 1980.

Hethcote, H.W. and Yorke, J.A., *Gonorrhea Transmission Dynamics and Control*, Lecture Notes in Biomathematics No. 56, Springer Verlag, Berlin, 1984.

Hethcote, H.W., Yorke, J.A. and Nold, A., "Gonorrhea modelling: a comparison of control methods", *Math. Biosci.*, 53, pages 93-109, 1982.

Hill, G.C.R., *The Mathematics of Epidemics*, University of Bristol Department of Engineering Mathematics, Undergraduate Dissertation, 1986.

Kemper, J.T., "On the identification of superspreaders for infectious diseases: a deterministic model", *Math. Biosci.*, 48, pages 111-127, 1980.

Knox, E.G., "A transmission model for AIDS", *Eur. Jour. Epidemiol.*, 2, pp 165-177, 1986.

Kramer, M.A. & Reynolds, G.H., "Evaluation of a gonorrhea vaccine and other gonorrhea control strategies based on computer simulation modelling", *Differential Equations and Applications in Ecology, Epidemics and Population Problems*, edited by Busenberg, S. and Cooke, K.L., Academic Press, New York, pages 97-114, 1981.

McManus, T.J. and McEvoy, M. "Some aspects of male homosexual behaviour in the United Kingdom", *Br. Jour. Sexual Med.*, April 1987, pages 110 et seq.

Mansfield, E. and Hensley, C. "The logistic process: tables of the stochastic epidemic curve and applications", *J. Roy. Stat. Soc.*, Series *B*, 22, pp 332-7, 1960.

May, R.M. & Anderson, R.M., "Transmission dynamics of HIV infection", *Nature*, 326, pp 137-142, 1987.

Peto, J. "AIDS and promiscuity", *Lancet*, 1986, ii, 979.

Reece, G., "Varieties of sexual contact", *Nature*, 327, p. 288, 1987.

Tovey, S.J. "Condoms and AIDS prevention", *Lancet*, 1987, *i*, 567.

Weber, J.N. and ten others "Human Immunodeficiency Virus infection in two cohorts of homosexual men: neutralising sera and association of anti-gag antibody with prognosis", *Lancet*, 1987, *i*, 119.

Williams, T. "The simple stochastic epidemic curve for large populations of susceptibles", *Biometrika*, 52, pp 571-9, 1965.

9 ACKNOWLEDGEMENTS

I should like to acknowledge the generous financial support of the Terrence Higgins Trust and the Aled Richards Trust.

I also wish to express my thanks to the large number of my colleagues and friends who have helped with the work described in this paper, including: Professor Tony Coxon, who helped with all the sociological aspects of the problem of modelling the spread of HIV; Dr Stuart Glover, who has explained to me many of the clinical aspects of HIV infection and its consequences; Professor Geoffrey Grimmett, who shared with me some of his profound understanding of stochastic processes; Dr Alfred Roome, for his advice on virology and for indicating many of the recent sources used here; my students Graham Hill, Chris Mitchell, Dan Morgan and Jon Smith, for their enthusiasm and skill.

STOCHASTIC PROCESS MODELS IN CLINICAL PSYCHOLOGY AND PSYCHIATRY

A. Pickles
(MRC Child Psychiatry Unit, Institute of Psychiatry, DeCrespigny Park, London)

and

R. Crouchley
(Department of Sociology, University of Surrey, Guildford)

ABSTRACT

The advantages of the use of models in the analysis of data are discussed and contrasted with more standard approaches. The use of models is illustrated in two examples; a Wiener process model of the durations of foster-placements and a multivariate extreme-value model of conduct problems among the children of psychiatric patients.

1. HYPOTHESIS TESTING VERSUS MODEL BUILDING

In psychology, as elsewhere, the application of statistics to the analysis of experimental results has undoubtedly led to better experimental design and more efficient testing of treatment effects. However, in practice it may also have tended to result in a narrowing of data analysis to one of testing for significant differences rather than with the broader concern to characterise the structure of the process under study. With this narrower conception of the objectives of an analysis, the choice of methods is often reduced to an almost exclusive consideration of the relative efficiencies of a parametric estimator and a non-parametric or partially parametric alternative. Where the relative loss of efficiency is small, the less parametric estimator will be preferred, since it usually requires fewer assumptions to be made about the structure of the data and the underlying process.

However, in many non-experimental situations the interest of the empirical researcher is focussed not only on the determination of significant sources of variation, but also on the gaining of some broader understanding of the process under study. For example, since survey data represent real-life processes there is a general interest in the results of an analysis as a source of process description. A statistical model of the process, even one that may make bold (but potentially testable) assumptions, is often more useful in this respect than a series of more agnostic hypothesis tests. A proper evaluation of such models inevitably requires the researcher to assess the plausability of the implied mechanisms; a task that can force valuable conceptual and theoretical clarification.

In some situations this concern with mechanism may be more highly focussed. In many studies the effects of a variable on an outcome might occur through one or more of several mechanisms, and corresponding to each may be differing degrees of opportunity for intervention and different treatments that may be appropriate. It is not only more useful, but considerably more persuasive to be able to show that not only is there a significant association between an explanatory variable and an outcome, but that it achieves its effect by one, hopefully theoretically more sensible mechanism, rather than another. We illustrate these points in Section 2 using, as an example, an analysis of foster placement data. Where current data is not sufficient to distinguish among mechanisms, explicit process models can help indicate the additional data required to achieve it.

In more complicated sample designs, such as the hierarchical sampling of children from within sampled classes from within sampled schools, correlation among the observations from within a sample unit may be expected. For outcomes on a continuous scale, a variety of methods is available to fit familiar regression models to such data [17]. For simple discrete outcome variables the usual models that are applied are threshold response models based on the normal or logistic distribution. The current methods for applying these models to data from complex designs are either computationally very burdensome or do not give estimates and tests for all the aspects of the process of interest. In Section 3 we examine this problem within an example of a longitudinal family study of child conduct disturbance. Some preliminary results are presented from the application of a multivariate threshold response model that is based on the extreme value distribution. This model is consistent with an onset mechanism associated with extreme stress. The model appears to possess considerable potential not only for longitudinal family study designs, such as that of the example, but also for ordinary panel studies and other studies with multiple indicators.

2. THE DURATION OF FOSTER PLACEMENTS

2.1 The Data

The data, from Hind [18], concern the foster placements of 90 children prepared for placement by the Barnardo's Pre-Fostering Unit. The data observation period included the start of each of these placements and covered the period from the end of 1978 to August 1984. Three forms of fostering outcome were possible. The first of these was where placement breakdown was observed (30). The second was where the child reached the age of legal independence (age 18) at which point the foster placement as a legal entity was terminated (1). The third was where the placement was still continuing at the end of the study (59).

The objective of the analysis was to determine the characteristics of the foster-family and the child, in particular their previous experience and preparation, that contributed to a positive outcome. The contending explanatory variables are listed in Table 1.

2.2 Proportional Hazards and Cox's Partial Likelihood

Hind chose to analyse these data using a proportional hazards survival (PH) model [9], the method which is now almost universally applied to duration data of almost any sort. In this context, those placements that end in breakdown are treated as 'failures', whilst the remainder are treated as 'censored' before failure could be observed, by some other process assumed independent. The impact of explanatory variables X_i is typically assumed to act multiplicatively on some baseline instantaneous risk of failure $\lambda_o(t)$, such that

$$\lambda_i(t) = \lambda_o(t)\exp(\beta X_i) \tag{2.2.1}$$

Parameter estimates and their standard errors can be obtained using partial likelihood [9, 10] within standard packages (e.g. GLIM using the macro of Clayton and Cuzick [8]). Based upon the ranks of the observed durations, this procedure allows a non-parametric representation of the baseline hazard.

Such an analysis is known to have high efficiency against simple parametric alternatives, such as the exponential and Weibull, and simple tests exist for the principal assumption of proportionality. Different baseline hazards may be allowed for using stratification and estimates of them are easily obtained (e.g. using Breslow Scores (see discussion in [9]). With such obvious advantages why use anything else?

Variable List

1.	PREP	length of preparation of the child in months
2.	SEX	1 = male, 2 = female
3.	ETH	1 = caucasian, 2 = non caucasian
4.	BEH	0 no behavioural problems 1 } 2 } number of behavioural problems 3 } 4 }
5.	EDUC	1 = child attends mainstream school 2 = child attends special school
6.	AGE	age at start of placement in months
7.	CARE	length of time the child has been in care expressed as a % of the child's chronological age
8.	MOVE	number of moves the child has experienced whilst being in care
9.	AGENCY	1 = foster family found by local authority 2 = foster family found by specialist agency
10.	EXPR	length of time the foster mother has previously acted in this capacity: 0 = never, 1 = under 1 year, 2 = 1-4 years, 3 = 4+ years
11.	CHILD	number of children within the foster home within 5 years of age of the foster child
12.	CONT	agreed level of contact between the child natural parents and the child during placement 1 once a month 2 once every 2 months 3 once every 3 months 4 once every 4-6 months 5 once every 6+ months 6 not at all

Table 1 Variable list and coding before standardization to zero mean and standard deviation one.

2.3 *Inverse Gaussian Models of Conciliation and Breakdown*

The results of an analysis using the PH model inform us about those measured variables that have an impact upon the relative risk of breakdown. But only in a quite limited sense do they advance our conceptualisation of the process of foster child-foster family interaction. Elevated risks may be identified but the risk mechanism is not elucidated. A parametric model based on some plausible theory might be more informative.

The foster child and family may be usefully conceived as engaged in continuous negotiation. Since we find it natural to speak metaphorically about negotiations in terms of the distance between the parties involved, a formal model based on such a dimension seems appropriate. In some contexts we can observe the variation in the distance directly (e.g. differences in offers and demands in wage negotiations) but this is not necessary for the estimation of a model. Where breakdown or conciliation are observed, the time to such events can be related to a time of transit from an initial separation distance to some threshold value. Thus strike durations might be related to initial differences in wage offer and demand.

At the start of the process the parties from foster family i may be separated by a distance a_i and breakdown occurs if this distance exceeds c_i. In fact we are concerned only with the separation distance relative to the threshold (c_i-a_i), say d_i. Without loss of generality we can take $d_i(t)$, the separation distance at time t, as equal to 0 at t=0, and the threshold to be at a distance γ_i from this. The simplest assumption we can make is that convergence or divergence of the parties occurs with a certain velocity but one that is subject to random fluctuation. If we assume that for any interval of time (t_1,t_2), $t_1 \geq 0, t_2 > t_1$, the distance traversed $d_i(t_1)-d_i(t_2)$ is normally distributed with

$$E[d(t_1)-d(t_2)] = \mu_i.(t_1-t_2), \qquad (2.3.1)$$

variance

$$\sigma_i^2.(t_1-t_2)$$

and that for non-overlapping intervals the distances traversed are independently distributed, then $d_i(t)$ is a Wiener process. The random variable s, the time taken for d_i to exceed the threshold, is the first passage time through a single absorbing barrier. This is known to possess an inverse Gaussian (IG) distribution (see, for example [11], Chapter 5), such that

$$g(s) = \gamma_i\sigma_i^{-1}(2\pi s^3)^{-1/2},\exp[-(\gamma_i-\mu_i s)^2(2\sigma_i^2 s)^{-1}] \quad (2.3.2)$$

The mean time to failure is, not surprisingly, equal to γ_i/μ_i, the initial distance from the threshold divided by the mean velocity. The variance of the time to failure is equal to $\gamma_i\sigma_i^2\mu_i^{-3}$ or to $(\gamma_i/\mu_i)^3(\sigma_i^2/\gamma_i^2)$. This latter form brings out the mean variance relationship that is emphasized in the use of the IG distribution in generalized linear models [22], with the variance being proportional to the mean cubed and the second term representing the scale parameter.

Unlike most other parametric survival time distributions (e.g. Weibull, Gompertz, gamma, lognormal) the IG may be defective, for the velocity of movement need not be towards the threshold at all, leading to the possibility that eventual breakdown is not inevitable. In addition, the hazard function need not be monotonic. Figure 1 shows such an IG hazard function form. In the context of fostering this may be important. It is commonly held that an early 'honeymoon' period is enjoyed at the start of foster placement resulting in a period of low risk of breakdown. There then follows a period of higher risk, seen as the period during which a more permanent relationship is worked out, which once negotiated is followed by a second period of low risk.

As with most multi-parameter distributions Equation (2.3.2) represents just one of several different parametrizations of the IG distribution. When the parameters themselves, or simple combinations of them, are made functions of explanatory variables, numerous alternative forms are possible. In most applications the mean duration (γ_i/μ_i) is equated to a linear predictor of explanatory variables, either directly [15] or using a log-link function to ensure positive fitted durations [14]. Where the distribution may be defective, implying an infinite mean, neither is altogether satisfactory. The canonical power link function (p22, [22]), with power minus half, gives an infinite fitted duration with a linear predictor of zero, but the linear predictor itself must be bounded to the right at zero.

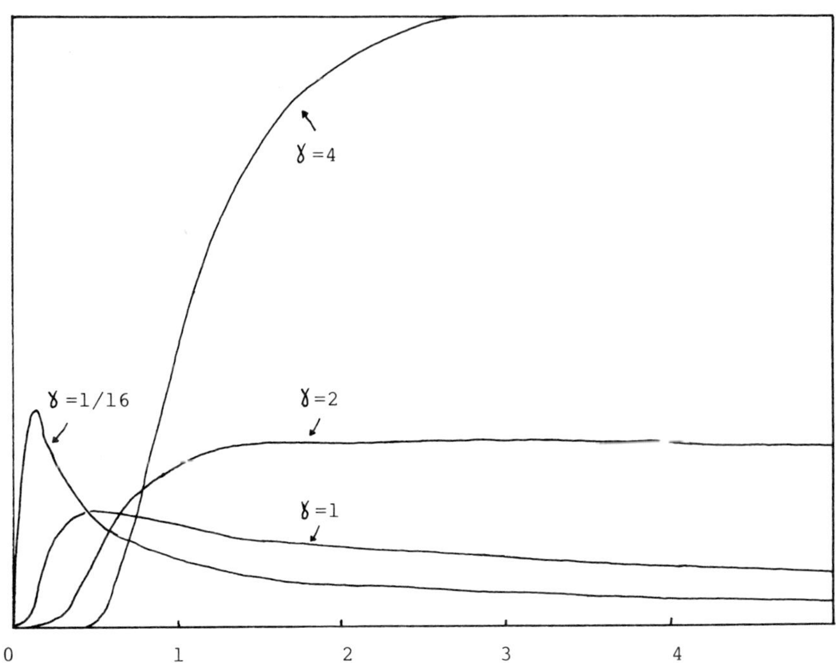

Fig. 1 Inverse Gaussian hazard-function for $\gamma/\mu = 1$

Normal linear theory allows the simultaneous use of several linear predictors in a relatively straightforward way (e.g. [17]) allowing the mean, the variance (or scale parameter) and even the coefficients to be modelled. The possibility of a second linear predictor with the IG distribution was suggested by Folks and Chhikura [15], who proposed choosing the inverse of the scale parameter (γ_i^2/σ_i^3).

Although following the tradition of modelling the mean and scale parameter of the survival distribution is clearly possible with the foster placement data, the likely occurrence of a defective distribution would have at least complicated the estimation procedure. In fact there is an alternative parameterization of the IG that is also a member of the exponential family, based upon μ_i/σ_i and γ_i/σ_i (p22 [12]). In the context of preparing children and parents for foster placement this parameterization looks more appealing. Rather than the explanatory variables influencing the expected duration directly, their impact may occur differentially on the initial distance or velocity. Preparation of the child is most likely to influence initial expectations, and thus the distance γ_i, whereas the greater maturity of adults would lead one to expect that the effects of their experience (or lack of it) would be exhibited over an extended period of time, and thus in the velocity μ_i. It is also possible for the same variable to influence both γ_i and μ_i. The parametrization chosen was

$$\gamma_i/\sigma_i = \exp(\underline{\alpha}'\underline{x}_i) \quad (2.3.3)$$

$$\mu_i/\sigma_i = \underline{\beta}'\underline{x}_i \quad (2.3.4)$$

This form is natural in that it ensures the appropriate constraints are met. It is of course recognized that the different functional forms for γ_i/σ_i and μ_i/σ_i are also necessary to ensure the separate identifiability of α and β.

2.4 A Comparison of Results

Tables 2 and 3 give the results obtained from the data for the PH and IG models respectively. The results

Variable	Parameters	Standard Errors
Constant	-0.352	-
PREP	0.095	0.209
SEX	0.070	0.218
ETH	0.167	0.226
BEH	-0.082	0.202
EDUC	-0.448	0.231
AGE	0.451	0.213
CARE	-0.508	0.252
MOVE	-0.067	0.248
AGENCY	-0.200	0.228
EXPR	-0.668	0.278
CHILD	0.178	0.253
CONT	0.188	0.217

Table 2 Parameter estimates and standard errors from Cox's partial likelihood proportional hazard model.

Variable	Parameter Estimates and χ^2 values					
	$\gamma_i = \exp(\underline{\alpha}'\underline{\chi}_i)$			$\mu_i = \underline{\beta}'\underline{\chi}_i$		
CONSTANT	α_1	0.094	-	β_1	-0.147	-
PREP	α_2	0.890	(1.47)	β_2	1.349	(0.67)
SEX	α_3	0.270	(3.28)	β_3	0.426	(2.61)
ETH	α_4	0.470	(1.92)	β_4	0.614	(5.54)
BEH	α_5	0.023	(0.03)	β_5	-0.184	(0.60)
EDUC	α_6	0.078	(0.38)	β_6	-0.273	(1.10)
AGE	α_7	0.499	(3.73)	β_7	1.088	(9.99)
CARE	α_8	0.009	(0.01)	β_8	-0.302	(1.38)
MOVE	α_9	0.074	(0.21)	β_9	0.025	(0.01)
AGENCY	α_{10}	0.099	(0.43)	β_{10}	-0.080	(0.13)
EXPR	α_{11}	-0.181	(1.64)	β_{11}	-0.647	(5.83)
CHILD	α_{12}	-0.596	(3.08)	β_{12}	-0.361	(1.65)
CONT	α_{13}	-0.081	(0.61)	β_{13}	-0.058	(0.09)

Log likelihood of the full model = -61.4344.

Critical values $\chi^2(1,0.05) = 3.84$, $\chi^2(1,0.10) = 2.71$.

Table 3 Inverse Gaussian parameter estimates and χ^2 tests in parentheses for removing each variable in turn with replacement.

provide examples of each of the effects described. Maternal experience, highly significant in the PH model, has its impact primarily through the β (velocity) coefficient of the IG model. Child preparation has no effect in the PH model but a slight hint of an effect through the α coefficient (distance) of the IG model. Both experience and preparation have effects in the expected direction (the poor performance of preparation may in part reflect that longer preparation may be associated with more disturbed or more 'difficult to place' children). Ethnicity, gives an insignificant increase in the PH hazard, whereas in the IG model it gives a significant β coefficient. Other similar aged children in the home have no effect according to the PH model but in the IG model appear to place the relationship closer to the threshold initially, possibly reflecting initial jealousy and rivalry. This is followed by a compensating effect, in terms of risk of breakdown, of a shift in the velocity away from the threshold, possibly reflecting the longer run positive value of a sib type relationship.

A direct comparison of the goodness-of-fit of two such different models is difficult. Figure 2 shows a Kaplan-Meier plot of the residuals from the models. Those for the IG model fall nicely on the 45 degree line whilst those for the PH model show a distinct curve, suggesting some mispecification.

Since the identifiability of the two linear predictors rests upon them having different link functions, it is reasonable to ask whether they really do add separate information to the analysis. Some dependence between the linear predictors can be seen in figure 3. The importance of this dependence for inference was investigated informally, considering the problem as similar to that of multi-collinearity in an ordinary regression model. Taking a model with no linear predictors, adding that for the velocity gives a chi-square improvement of 18.3, followed by a further improvement of 9.6 on adding that for the threshold distance. Reversing the order of addition gives 10.9 for threshold distance and 17.0 for velocity. The relative stability of the chi-squares attributed to each linear predictor gives some support to our view that separate effects are indicated.

A more extensive discussion of the results can be found elsewhere [13].

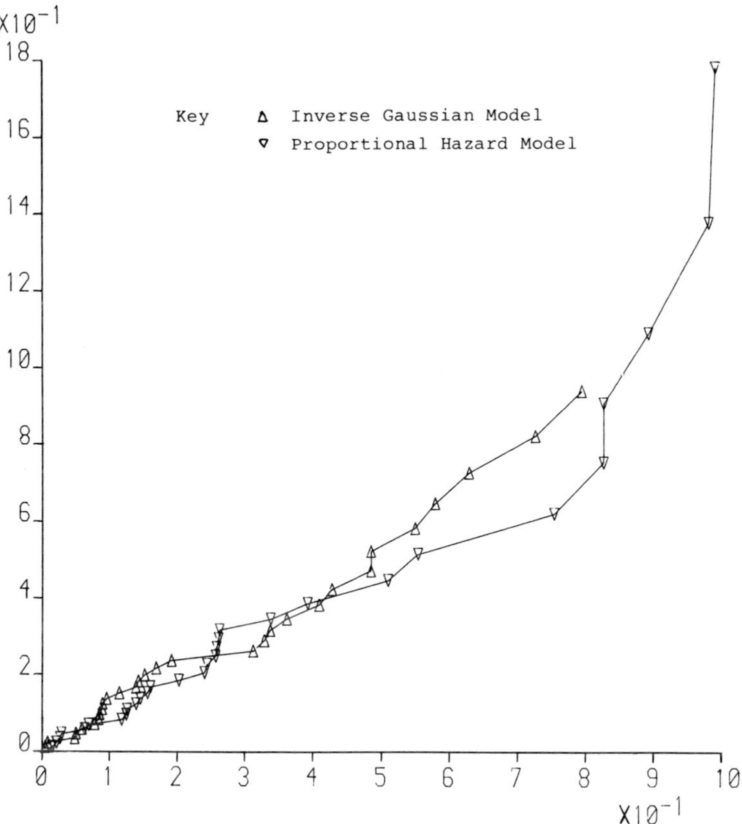

Fig. 2 Kaplan-Meier plot of residuals from the proportional hazard and inverse Gaussian models.

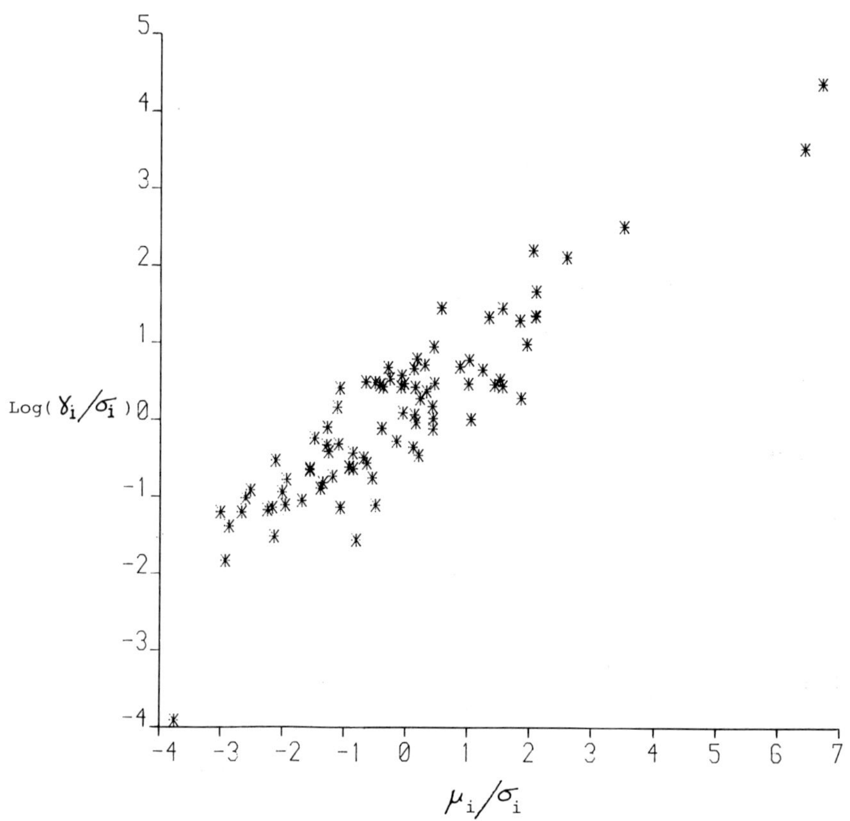

Fig. 3 Plot of estimated velocities and thresholds from the inverse Gaussian model.

3. LONGITUDINAL FAMILY STUDIES

Research in child psychiatry is frequently concerned to examine the processes of onset and maintenance of child disorder in the context of the family genetic and social environment. The design of such studies often involves the sampling and subsequent observation of all the children within families that are thought to be at risk. The data for the second example of this paper comes from the Family Illness study of Rutter and Quinton [25]. This study followed over a five year period the families of parents, at least one of whom had recently been a psychiatric patient. A major interest was to determine whether the mechanism for the increased risk of behavioural disturbance (measured as a binary variable) that such children exhibit lay in having a psychiatrically disturbed parent or in the exposure to marital discord and breakdown that often accompanies it. The major statistical complication introduced by this design is the inevitable correlation among sibs in the error term of any model. Child based analyses that ignore intra-family correlation typically exaggerate the effect and significance of family level variables.

A natural model for the analysis of the duration until onset of behavioural disturbance in the children would be a multivariate form of the PH model. Estimation of such a model, extending the partial likelihood approach to sets of non-independent survival times, has been attempted in the case of the survival times of fathers and their sons, but has not yet proved tractable in general [6, 7].

3.2 *Threshold Response Models*

An alternative approach is to recast the problem in discrete time as panel data. With interval level response measures a range of commonly used models are available from simple dummy variable 'within' estimators to repeated measures ANOVA, more general variance components analysis, or if very weak assumptions about the correlation structure are required, MANOVA. However, much data relating to onset is, as here, of a discrete form, often of the binary response - well or ill. The principles underlying these methods for interval level responses can be carried forward into the realm of discrete response variables by assuming that these responses arise from a continuously distributed latent variable that is observed only in a discrete form as it falls above or below some threshold value.

The continuous response variable Y^*_{jkt}, of child $k, (k = 1,\ldots,n_j)$, from family $j, (j = 1,\ldots,J)$ at time $t, (t = 1,\ldots,T)$ is defined by the regression relationship.

$$Y^*_{jkt} = \beta' x_{jkt} + u_{jkt} \qquad (3.2.1)$$

In practice we observe only the (0,1) binary variable Y_{jkt} defined by whether Y^*_{jkt} is below or above a threshold of zero. We therefore obtain

$$\begin{aligned}\text{Prob}[Y_{jkt} = 1] &= \text{Prob}[u_{jkt} > -\beta' x_{jkt}] \\ &= 1 - F(-\beta' x_{jkt}) \qquad (3.2.2) \\ &= 1 - F(-\eta_{jkt})\end{aligned}$$

where F(.) is the c.d.f. of the 'regression' error u_{jkt}.

An assumption of the familiar normal error leads to a probit model [16] of the form

$$\text{Prob}(Y_{jkt} = 1] = 1 - \int_{-\infty}^{-\eta_{jkt}/\sigma} (2\pi)^{-1/2} \exp(u^2/2)\,du \qquad (3.2.3)$$

The logistic density has a particularly simple c.d.f. that gives the familiar logit model

$$\text{Prob}[Y_{jkt} = 1] = \exp(\eta_{jkt})/[1+\exp(\eta_{jkt})] \qquad (3.2.4)$$

The less familiar extreme value (EV) distribution also has a simple c.d.f. that gives

$$\text{Prob}[Y_{jkt} = 1] = 1-\exp[-\exp(\eta_{jkt})] \qquad (3.2.5)$$

the complementary log-log model.

All three are standard models within the computer package GLIM [3] and McCullagh and Nelder [22] show that, when appropriately standardized, their c.d.f.s differ only in the tails. The complementary log-log has found occasional use as a model of a partially observed event process (e.g. [24]) but rarely elsewhere. However, in the context of our application it seemed an attractive choice. A plausible model of the onset of psychiatric disorder (at least for some affective disorders such as depression) is that it is provoked by the occurrence of an extreme stress, beyond that which the individual can manage. Thus our concern is focussed upon whether, during the period of interest, the most extreme stress experienced fell below the threshold and thus within the range of manageability. The probit model, viewed from a similar standpoint, would suggest that thresholds and/or stressful environments are normally distributed, the result of the addition of a large number of contributing effects. By contrast, the complementary log-log suggests that conditional on knowledge of the most extreme event, the occurrence during this period of more minor stressful events is irrelevant. Of course, in the absence of detailed information about all stressful events, the similarities of the normal and extreme-value of c.d.f.'s would make the task of empirically distinguishing the two models difficult.

3.3 Multivariate Threshold Response Models

Because of the correlation across both time and sibs, the responses $\{Y_{jkt}\}$ will not be independent. However, under random sampling of families, independent response vectors, each with $T \times n_j$ elements can be obtained, but these will require analysis using a multivariate response model. We considered the extension of the three threshold response models to the multivariate context.

3.3.1 Logit Model and Conditional Likelihood

A general multivariate logistic distribution does not exist, but some progress can be made if we are willing to assume structure to the pattern of correlations. If we assume that the correlations arise from the existence of time constant child and family effects the model may be specified by including dummy variables within the linear predictor for the response of each child

$$\eta_{jkt} = \alpha_{jk}+\alpha_j+\beta' x_{jkt} \qquad (3.3.1.1)$$

the logistic regression errors then being independent between children. But unlike the equivalent dummy variable model in linear regression, ordinary ML estimation of this model would lead to inconsistent estimates of the βs, owing to the 'incidental parameter problem' [23]

Where all the included covariates are strictly exogeneous [4] a conditional likelihood [2] may be formed, that eliminates the incidental parameters, the dummy variables $\{\alpha_{jk}, \alpha_j\}$, by conditioning on their sufficient statistics, $\tau_{jk} = \Sigma_t Y_{jkt}$ and $\tau_j = \Sigma_k \Sigma_t Y_{jkt}$. Maximising this conditional likelihood can yield surprisingly efficient estimates of structural parameters (and standard errors) without any need to make assumptions as to the distribution of the incidental parameters. However, the sufficient statistics for these incidental parameters are often also sufficient for many of the effects of interest in the model. We therefore do not pursue this further.

3.3.2 *The Multivariate Probit Model*

Unlike the logit model, sufficient statistics do not exist for the incidental parameters of equation (3.3.1.1) in the linear predictor of a probit model. Conditional estimation of the structural parameters is therefore not possible. However, the multivariate probit [1], being based on the multivariate normal (MVN) distribution, is theoretically capable of incorporating the desired correlation structure directly within the model. Considering just the case of only children with two response periods, calculations for the likelihood of the observed response vector take the form of

$$\text{Prob}[Y_{j11} = 0, Y_{j12} = 0] = F(-\eta_{j11}, -\eta_{j12})$$

$$= \int_{-\infty}^{-\eta_{j11}} \int_{-\infty}^{-\eta_{j12}} f(u_{j11}, u_{j12})\, d(u_{j11}, u_{j12}) \qquad (3.3.2.1)$$

where f(.,.) is a bivariate normal density with an estimated covariance matrix

$$\begin{bmatrix} 1 & \rho^2 \\ \rho^2 & 1 \end{bmatrix}$$

The extension to additional responses is straightforward.

Unfortunately, the necessary integration must be performed numerically, and this imposes strict practical limitations. Approximation methods, such as that of Clark [5], have been used to solve problems requiring up to ten dimensions, but the computational task remains substantial and performance uncertain [19].

3.3.3 *The Multivariate Extreme Value Model*

Various forms of the multivariate extreme value distribution have been proposed (chapter 42 [21]; [26]) and few have yet to receive serious consideration from applied statisticians. Preliminary consideration suggested that the form proposed by Gumble [20] (Johnson and Kotz - type B) offered potential. With this distribution the vector response probability of the previous section becomes

$$\mathrm{Prob}[Y_{j11} = 0, Y_{j12} = 0] = G(-\eta_{j11}, -\eta_{j12})$$
$$= \exp[-\{\exp(m.\eta_{j11}) + \exp(m.\eta_{j12})\}^{1/m}] \qquad (3.3.3.1)$$

with the corresponding correlation between the errors being given by

$$\rho = 1 - m^{-2} \; (m \geq 1) \qquad (3.3.3.2)$$

Thus a bivariate threshold response model based on the bivariate EV distribution is hardly more complex than the univariate. Moreover, further responses may be included and still the integration remains analytically tractable and thus computationally fast.

Although the obvious multivariate generalizations of the EV distribution do not possess the completely general covariance structure of the MVN, they can often be structured to match that of the data at hand. For the family illness data we can expect a high positive correlation over time in the responses of each child arising partly from time constant omitted variables describing the propensity of the child to conduct disorder, and secondly from an expectation of continuity in the pattern of family interaction in which different children may be exposed to or even the focus of family stress. A positive correlation can also be expected across sibs arising from the various omitted variables describing the family environment in which they live and the differing sensitivities that they may share, for example by genetic inheritance. This kind of hierarchical structure is shown in Figure 4.

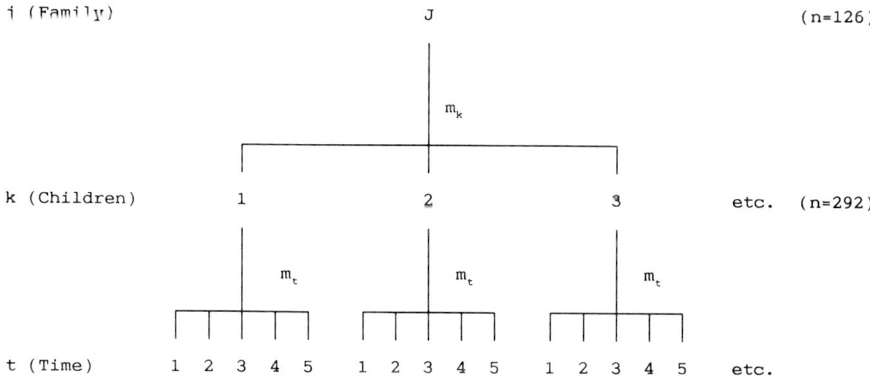

Fig. 4 Hierarchical correlation structure for longitudinal family study.

A multivariate EV model reflecting this pattern is given by

$$F(\{Y_{jkt}=0\},k=1,\ldots,n_j;t=1,\ldots,T)$$

$$= \exp\left[-\sum_{k=1}^{n_j}\left[\{\sum_{t=1}^{T}\exp(m_t.\eta_{jkt})\}^{m_k/m_t}\right]^{1/m_k}\right] \quad (3.3.3.3)$$

with $m_t \geq m_k \geq 1$.

3.4 Results from the Multivariate Extreme Value Model

The model of equation (3.3.3.3) was applied to the nine element vector response process defined by the responses from the first three years of the study data for up to three children from each family. The explanatory variables used in this preliminary application of the model are described in Table 4.

The parameter estimates and test statistics are given in Table 5 for models which assume all the child observations are independent, allow for within child correlation but not within family, and for the full model with both.

The residual correlation over time in responses is clearly substantial and the inclusion of this correlation in the model substantially reduces the magnitude and significance of the explanatory variables. The correlation between children of the same family is relatively small, but even so its inclusion substantially reduces the likelihood ratio test statistic for the impact of parental personality disorder. The final model suggests that both parental psychiatric condition and marital discord result in behavioural disturbance in the children, through the evidence for the effects of marital discord are more marginal. The greater impact of marital discord on boys found by Rutter and Quinton [25] is consistent with the parameter estimates obtained, although this difference is not significant within this analysis. The effect of psychiatric disorder is also rather larger here.

Response Variable	Codes
CHILD B-SCORE	1 = teacher rating of child classified as conduct or mixed disorder 0 = other
CHILD A-SCORE	as B-Score but rated by parent
Explanatory Variables	
1. SEX	Sex of child 0 = boy, 1 = girl
2. MARITAL DISCORD IN YEAR, t	0 = marriage non-discordant 1 = discordant or broken marriage
3. PARENT	0 = neither parent personality disordered at time 0 1 = one or both parents personality disordered at time 0
4. CLASS	Social class of family

Table 4 Variables in the Family Illness Example

Coefficient	Independence	Correlated Time Only	Correlated Child and Time
Constant	-2.682	-2.614	-2.566
Sex	0.147	0.062	0.130
Discord	1.056	0.756	0.761
Sex Discord	-0.902	-0.589	-0.629
Parent	0.778	0.874	0.735
Time Correlation	0.000	0.548	0.555
Child Correlation	0.000	0.000	0.060
Log-Likelihood	-173.78	-162.37	-161.37
Likelihood Ratio Tests			
Sex Discord (1df)	2.90	1.38	1.62
Discord + Sex Discord (2df)	9.28	4.94	4.90
Parent (1df)	9.30	6.58	4.02

Table 5 Parameter estimates and significance tests for the multivariate extreme value threshold response model.

3.5 Further Developments

Several extensions to this initial application of the multivariate EV model are possible.

Extending the response vector to include more children from the larger families or further periods of response is computationally straightforward. However, preliminary tests suggested that their inclusion made the likelihood maximisation more diffult. Faster convergence, indeed a better model, may require the within family correlation to vary with family size. The linking of the correlation parameters to covariates may also be useful in examining how the continuity in responses over time varies across individuals.

The response vector need not include a single repeated measure, but may be made up of several different indicators. We illustrate this within our example by supplementing the teacher ratings of child behaviour (Rutter B-score) by parental ratings (Rutter A-score). Table 6 presents results for data from a single period and up to 4 sibs. The low residual correlation across measures is characteristic, and

Coefficient		Parameter Estimate
Constant		-0.774
Sex		-0.406
Discord		1.221
Discord Sex		0.305
Parent on B		0.326
Parent on A		0.181
Class on A		-0.026
Indicator Correlation		0.710
Child Correlation		0.707
Likelihood Ratio Tests		
Discord+sex Discord	(2df)	2.65
Parent on A and B	(2df)	3.99
Class on A	(-df)	0.21

Table 6 Parameter estimates and significance tests for two indicator multivariate extreme value threshold response model.

seems to arise in part from the way children behave differently in the home than at school, so-called situational effects, as well as more general measurement problems. Note that with two response indicators the function of the regression covariates is more complicated, representing either their impact upon the latent variable defined by the indicators and/or the sytematic differences in measurement error of the indicators. We have illustrated examples of various kinds. First the sex and discord effects are estimated as common to both indicators. The effects of parent disorder have been allowed to differ, though the estimated effects are not significantly different from one another or from zero. Finally, the social class covariate has been included only on the A-score linear predictor to examine, for example, whether teachers systematically rated lower class children poorly or whether lower class parents possessed lower behavioural expectations for their children. The parameter estimate suggests no such effect.

ACKNOWLEDGEMENTS

We would like to thank Greg Hind for providing the fostering data and David Quinton for providing the family psychiatric data used in the analyses. Richard Smith provided valuable discussion.

REFERENCES

[1] Aitchison, J. and Bennett, J. (1970), "Polychotomous Quantal Response by Maximum Indicant", *Biometrika*, **57**, 253-62.

[2] Anderson, E.B., (1970), "Asymptotic Properties of Conditional Maximum Likelihood Estimators", *Journal of the Royal Statistical Society B*, **32**, 283-301.

[3] Baker, R.J. and Nelder, J.A., (1978), "The GLIM System: Release 3. Generalised Linear Interactive Models", Numerical Algorithms Group, Oxford.

[4] Chamberlain, G., (1985), "Heterogeneity, Omitted Variable Bias, and Duration Dependence", In Eds. J.J. Heckman and B. Singer, "Longitudinal Analysis of Labor Market Data", Cambridge University Press, Cambridge, 3-38.

[5] Clark, C., (1961), "The Greatest of a Finite Set of Random Variables", *Operational Research*, **9**, 145-62.

[6] Clayton, D., (1978), "A Model for Association in Bivariate Life-tables and its Application in Epidemiological Studies of Familial Tendency in Chronic Diseases", *Biometrika*, **65**, 141-51.

[7] Clayton, D. and Cuzick, J., (1985), "Multivariate Generalizations of the Proportional Hazards Model", *Journal of the Royal Statistical Society,* A**148**, 82-117.

[8] Clayton, D. and Cuzick, J., (1985), "The EM Algorithm for Cox's Regression Model using GLIM", Applied Statistics, **34**, 148-57.

[9] Cox, D.R., (1972), "Regression Models and Life-tables (with discussion)", *Journal of the Royal Statistical Society B,* **74**, 187-220.

[10] Cox, D.R., (1975), "Partial Likelihood", Biometrika **62**, 296-76.

[11] Cox, D.R. and Miller, H.D., (1965), "The Theory of Stochastic Processes", Mathuen, London.

[12] Cox, D.R. and Oakes, D., (1984), "Analysis of Survival Data", Chapman and Hall, London.

[13] Crouchley, R., (1987), "The Inverse Gaussian Probability Distribution as a Model for the Duration of a two-sided Bargaining Process", Mimeo. Dept. of Sociology, University of Surrey.

[14] Davies, R.B. and Pickles, A.R., (1987), "A Joint Trip Timing Store-Type Choice Model for Grocery Shopping, Including Inventory Effects and Non-parametric Control for Omitted Variables", Transportation Research, **21**, A, 345-61.

[15] Folks, J.L. and Chhikara, R.S., (1987), "The Inverse Gaussian Distribution and Its Statistical Application - a Review", *Journal of the Royal Statistical Society, B,* **49**, 1-39.

[16] Goldberger, A.S., (1964), "Econometric Theory", Wiley, New York.

[17] Goldstein, H., (1987), "Multilevel Models in Educational and Social Research", Griffin, London.

[18] Hind, G., (1985), "Survival or Disruption", Unpublished MSc Dissertation, Dept. of Sociology, University of Surrey.

[19] Horowitz, J.L., Sparmann, J.M. and Daganzo, C.F., (1982), "An Investigation of the Accuracy of the Clark Approximation For the Multinomial Probit Model", Transportation Science, **16**, 382-401.

[20] Gumbel, E.J., (1960), "Distributions des Valeurs Extremes en Plusieurs Dimension", Publ. Inst. Statist. Univers. Paris, **9**, 171-173.

[21] Johnson, N.L. and Kotz, S., (1972), "Distributions in Statistics: Continuous Multivariate Distributions", Wiley, New York.

[22] McCullagh, P. and Nelder, J.A., (1983), "Generalized Linear Models", Chapman and Hall, London.

[23] Neyman, J. and Scott, E.L., (1948), "Consistent Estimates Based on Partially Consistent Observations", *Econometrica*, **16**, 1-32.

[24] Pickles, A.R. and O'Farrell, P.N., (1987), "An analysis of Entrepreneurial Behaviour from Male Work Histories", Regional Studies, **21**, 425-44.

[25] Rutter, M. and Quinton, D., (1984), "Parental Psychiatric Disorder: Effects on Children, Psychological Medicine, **14**, 853-880.

[26] Smith, R.L., Tawn, J.J. and Yeun, H.K., (1988), "Statistics of Multivariate Extremes", Mimeo. Dept. of Mathematics, University of Surrey.

ESTIMATION AFTER STOPPING A CLINICAL TRIAL EARLY

M. D. Hughes and S. J. Pocock
*(Medical Statistics Unit,
London School of Hygiene and Tropical Medicine)*

SUMMARY

There is increasing emphasis on estimation of treatment effects in the medical literature. Many randomized clinical trials are now designed to allow for early termination if there is strong evidence of a treatment difference. However estimates obtained after the use of these stopping rules are overestimates, in expectation, of the true treatment difference. Using simulation of a placebo-controlled trial of a thrombolytic agent we describe the degree of bias in estimation that can be expected from the use of group sequential designs. On average, the bias is relatively small. More importantly, though, estimates arising from trials that stop early are necessarily large and lack precision. Classical methods of bias adjustment only have a minor effect on such estimates. We describe an alternative, Bayesian, approach which produces more plausible estimates of effect.

1. INTRODUCTION

The ethical desirability of stopping a clinical trial early if one treatment is shown, beyond reasonable doubt, to be better than the alternative being studied is well recognised. Thus, many clinical trials in which patients are entered over a long period of time are subjected to interim analyses of the accumulating data. Stopping rules have been formulated [1,2,3] for such analyses so that the overall type 1 error is preserved at some level, e.g. 5%. These define a critical value for the test statistic (or, equivalently a nominal P-value) after each group of patients have been followed up with stopping of the trial if the statistic exceeds this value. However, the observed difference in treatment efficacy obtained for sequentially designed trials is an overestimate, in expectation, of the true underlying effect. Using simulation of a particular trial with which we have been involved, we shall describe the levels of bias that can arise and then suggest how prior belief of treatment effect can be used to produce more plausible estimates of effect particularly when stopping early.

2. A TRIAL WITH INTERIM ANALYSES

The APSAC Intervention Mortality Study (AIMS) [4] was designed to assess the effect on survival of a new thrombolytic therapy, APSAC, compared with placebo in patients with acute myocardial infarction. Patients were randomised and received one of the two treatments within six hours of the onset of symptoms. The survival curve for this disease shows a sharp initial fall within a few days of the infarct and then flattens out; the primary endpoint was therefore taken as mortality within 30 days which was expected to be about 12% on placebo. The trial was designed to have a maximum of 1000 patients on each of the active treatment and placebo with interim analyses carried out after 250, 500 and 750 patients had been allocated to each treatment and followed up for 30 days. Thus this was a four-group sequential design.

In order to illustrate some of the determinants of estimation bias we shall compare two different stopping rules in the context of the AIMS trial. Firstly, a rule described by O'Brien and Fleming [2] and the one actually used in the trial. This is characterized by an increasing sequence of nominal P-values making it difficult to stop at the first analysis unless there is a very extreme difference between the two treatments. In contrast, the second rule is a sequence of constant nominal P-values [1], which therefore makes stopping early comparatively easier. We have also simulated a trial with a fixed sample size and no interim analyses; estimates from this trial should exhibit no bias and so can be used as a benchmark for comparisons. Each of these three designs requires a different sample size in order to detect a particular treatment effect with a given power. The AIMS trial, in practice, had 80% power to detect a change in 30-day mortality rates from 12% to 8.2%. Therefore, in order to make valid comparisons, all the designs simulated have sample sizes based on this power calculation. Table 1 summarizes the designs giving both the sample size and the sequence of P-values used.

Design	Nominal P-values for significance at 5% level for analysis				Maximum sample size
	1	2	3	4	
1. O'Brien & Fleming stopping rule	0.0001	0.004	0.019	0.043	1000
2. Fixed nominal value stopping rule	0.018	0.018	0.018	0.018	1174
3. Fixed sample size	0.05	-	-	-	975

Table 1. Summary of trial designs simulated

For simplicity, in the simulations we have assumed that patients enter the trial in pairs and are randomised one each to the active treatment and placebo. After the appropriate number of patients have been entered, an analysis is conducted using an uncorrected chi-squared test. This is a two-sided test though our results will only consider differences in favour of the active treatment. The risk ratio (the ratio of the mortality rate for the active treatment to that for placebo) is estimated after stopping the trial either at an interim analysis according to the specified rule or at the final analysis. Thus a risk ratio of 100% represents no treatment difference and smaller ratios represent beneficial treatment effects compared with placebo.

3. ESTIMATION BIAS

For various specified underlying mortality rates for the active treatment, we now assess the influence of the design adopted on the sampling distribution of the observed risk ratio. Because the risk ratio is bounded below by zero this distribution is skew even for the fixed sample size design. Therefore in table 2 we give the median and 10% - 90% centile range for the distribution based upon 10000 simulations for each of the several assumed underlying rates. Median bias can therefore be evaluated by looking at the difference between the true risk ratio and the median obtained in the simulations. Obviously, the fixed sample size design shows no median bias. In contrast, both of the group sequential designs produce biassed estimates except in the case where there is no true difference between the active treatment and placebo. However the median bias is relatively small in all cases.

True risk ratio	Design		
	O'Brien & Fleming stopping rule	Fixed nominal value stopping rule	Fixed sample size
100%	100.00 85.60, 116.96	100.00 85.49, 116.93	100.00 85.59, 116.98
90%	89.91 75.61, 105.49	89.84 73.65, 104.35	90.00 76.27, 105.56
80%	79.84 64.56, 94.49	79.36 60.00, 93.08	80.00 67.46, 94.55
66.67%	65.38 51.32, 79.17	63.64 47.22, 77.54	66.67 55.65, 79.44
50%	49.21 36.55, 61.33	48.00 34.21, 60.81	50.00 40.68, 60.50

Table 2 Observed risk ratios: median and (10 - 90)% centile ranges by true risk ratio.

Using the centile range for the fixed size design as a benchmark, the increased skewness of the sampling distribution for the group sequential designs can be seen. An important feature to note is that both the skewness and the median bias is increased when the underlying risk ratio is of a size that the trial has a reasonable power to detect (the trials all have just over 80% power to detect a risk ratio of 66.67%). Comparing the two group sequential designs, it can be seen that bias is increased for designs that allow early stopping more readily: for all true risk ratios below 100%, the corresponding medians and centile points are all smaller for the fixed nominal value stopping rule than the O'Brien and Fleming rule.

It is useful to examine observed effects obtained from trials stopping at different stages. Restricting our attention just to the O'Brien and Fleming rule, table 3 shows the observed effects obtained from trials stopping at one of the first three analyses reporting a significant effect in favour of the active treatment, and also from trials continuing to the fourth and final analysis. Omitted from this table are the effects observed from a very small percentage of trials that stopped early favouring placebo (this is only 1% when the true risk ratio is 100%).

True risk ratio	Stage of stopping 1	2	3	4
100%	- - (0%)	58.33 52.17, 61.50 (0.2%)	69.74 65.57, 72.22 (0.8%)	100.00 86.13, 116.35 (98.0%)
90%	- - (0%)	57.05 52.78, 59.49 (1.0%)	68.37 62.97, 71.15 (4.7%)	90.98 78.57, 105.88 (94.2%)
80%	29.17 25.64, 34.04 (0.0%)	55.07 49.28, 59.15 (4.6%)	66.67 60.20, 70.19 (15.6%)	82.76 72.66, 96.03 (79.8%)
66.67%	27.50 22.11, 33.33 (0.0%)	52.31 44.28, 56.72 (22.2%)	63.74 56.76, 68.42 (38.2%)	74.34 66.37, 84.76 (39.3%)
50%	24.32 18.85, 29.08 (3.6%)	46.15 36.53, 53.33 (64.3%)	57.30 49.45, 64.38 (28.5%)	66.02 58.35, 73.61 (3.7%)

Table 3. Observed risk ratios: median and (10 - 90)% centile ranges (percentage of trials stopping) by stage of stopping for the O'Brien and Fleming design.

Clear from this table is the difficulty of stopping at the first interim analysis particularly for any realistic treatment effect. Looking down the columns relating to particular analyses, it is also clear that the median observed risk ratio changes little compared with the true underlying effect. A similar look at the 90% centile shows even less dependence on the true effect, which reflects the need to achieve a minimum risk ratio in the observed sample in order to stop at a particular interim analysis. Note, though, that this minimum is not a strict limit as we are also using the sample to give an estimate of the variance rather than using the true value. Thus, with early stopping, the observed effect bears little relation to the underlying risk ratio particularly when it is of moderate size. Also notable is that almost all trials that stop at either of the first two analyses necessarily underestimate the risk ratio. In contrast, trials that continue to the final analysis tend to produce overestimates of the true ratio.

The association between degree of bias and the proportion of trials stopping at each interim analysis is notable. For small treatment effects (e.g. a risk ratio of 80%) or large ones (e.g. 50%) the majority of trials stop at one particular analysis (the fourth and second, respectively) and there is little overall bias; for intermediate effects (e.g. 66.67%) there is a more varied distribution of stopping points and this results in increased bias. Thus in attempting to "sensitise" a trial to detect a given size of effect with reasonable power, we are removing the ability of the trial to estimate that size.

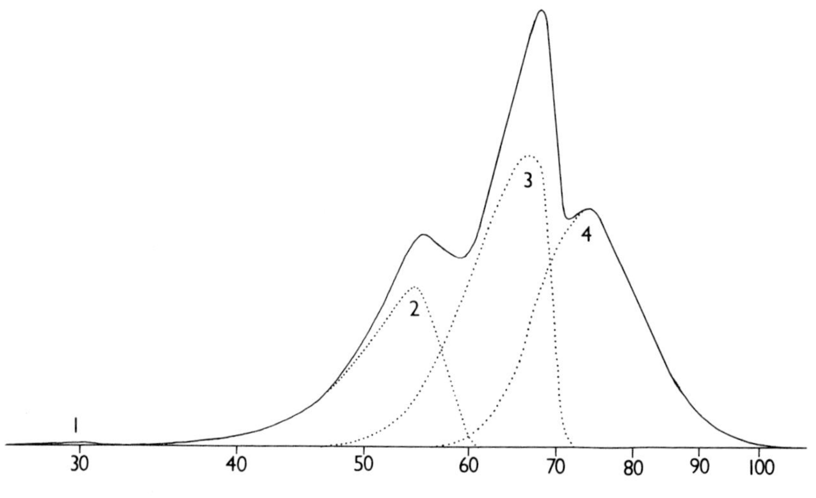

Fig. 1 Sampling distribution of observed risk ratio showing the contributions of each stopping point. (O'Brien and Fleming design; true risk ratio = 66.67%).

It is interesting to look at the actual shape of the sampling distribution. Figure 1, based upon 50000 simulations, shows how this distribution is composed of the distributions obtained at the first, second, third and fourth interim analyses when the true risk ratio is 66.67%. The areas under the curves of the component distributions are in proportion to the numbers of trials stopping at the appropriate stage. The increased steepness of the upper side of the third component distribution compared with the second is a reflection on the increased precision in the estimate of variance used in the test statistic given the larger sample size available later in the trial. The multimodalities are the dominant characteristic of the summed sampling distribution, there being one peak for each possible analysis. The peak at about the true underlying ratio (66.67%) is somewhat fortuitous and examples can be readily found where the design imposes a trough at the true value! One consequence of this heterogeneity is that classes of effect may be deduced from results of several trials using the same design when in fact there is a common underlying true effect. This may be of relevance when undertaking an overview of several trials of a common therapy when group sequential designs have been used.

4. USING PRIOR INFORMATION TO ADJUST ESTIMATES

The previous section attempted to describe the characteristics of estimates arising from sequentially designed trials; the results presented are generalizable to other stopping rules, more or fewer interim analyses and to parameters other than the risk ratio. We now return to the AIMS trial more specifically and the results obtained from it.

The trial was stopped after the second interim analysis had been undertaken. 502 patients had been randomised to each treatment with 61 (12.2%) deaths within 30 days on placebo compared with 32 (6.4%) on APSAC. The chi-squared test gave a nominal P-value of 0.002, less than 0.004 necessary for stopping. The observed risk ratio is 52.5% (95% confidence interval 34.8% to 79.0%). From a classical sampling point of view, this estimate, as we have seen from table 2, is biased but the level of bias is small. Thus methods of bias adjustment that have been proposed [5,6] only make a relatively small correction (of the order of a few percentage points) to the observed ratio. The reason for this becomes clear when we look at table 3. Whilst a true value of 66.67% gives rise to observed ratios of about 52.5% at the second analysis, the probability of stopping at that analysis for such a true value is small compared with later analyses. Effectively, the potential of data that might have been collected (and therefore the possibility of stopping at a later analysis) carries so much weight compared with the data actually accrued up until an early analysis that adjustment for bias is small.

For the clinical reader of a report from a trial that stopped early, such as from the AIMS trial, the observed treatment effect will almost certainly give a feeling of implausibility. Similarly, the statistician should also feel uneasy for two reasons:

(i) The observed treatment effect is necessarily large in order that the trial be terminated: how large is determined by the somewhat arbitrary choice of stopping rule that was made and so bears little relationship to the true effect;

(ii) the estimate obtained is of reduced precision because of the reduced sample size achieved.

Thus the clinician sees a result that is not consistent with his prior belief about the possible sizes of therapeutic effect that might realistically be expected, and the statistician might feel that treatment effects should be adjusted to reflect the reduced precision that allows, more readily, for the inflated estimates necessary for stopping. For both, a solution would be to apply Bayes Theorem and so use our prior belief of treatment effect to produce an adjusted "shrunken" estimate of treatment effect. In doing so the reduced precision of smaller amounts of data from early analyses is inherently catered for. We shall use the AIMS trial as an illustration of how this might be used in practice.

Maintaining our interest in the risk ratio, we felt that the following log-normal distribution described our prior belief for this parameter reasonably well:

$$\ln\,(\text{risk ratio}) \sim N(r,d^2) \tag{1}$$

where r was taken as ln(0.8) = -0.223 and d as 0.15. Thus the average effect is a risk ratio of 80%. 6.8% of the prior distribution lies above 100% whilst about 10% lies below 66.67% (reflecting a one-third reduction in mortality). This was developed mainly using information from earlier trials of similar thrombolytic therapies. These suggested risk ratios of about 80%. However, the possibility of an increased risk of bleeding problems associated with such therapies could theoretically lead to an increase in the risk ratio above 100% for patients receiving active treatment rather than placebo. On the other hand, APSAC was felt to be a more advanced derivative of earlier therapies and so might reduce mortality even further. The distribution of the observed risk ratio is given, approximately, by

$$\ln(\hat{\pi}_T/\hat{\pi}_P)\ \big|\pi_T,\pi_P \sim N\left[\ln(\pi_T/\pi_P),\ \frac{1-\pi_T}{n\pi_T}+\frac{1-\pi_P}{n\pi_P}\right] \tag{2}$$

where π_T and π_P are the true mortality rates on the active treatments and placebo, respectively, and $\hat{\pi}_T$ and $\hat{\pi}_P$ are assumed to be independent. This latter assumption could break down when stopping very close to the nominal P-value since this may impose a conditional relationship between the two observed rates. In this case simulation methods could be used as a check. Bayes Theorem is then applied using (1) and (2). This requires numerical integration though a very close approximation, particularly for largish sample sizes, can be found by using the observed mortality rates in the variance in (2) and using the standard result of Bayes Theorem applied to normal distributions with known variances. For the AIMS trial this gives a normal posterior distribution for the logged risk ratio with mean -0.37 and standard deviation 0.12. Taking the exponential of the mean gives a point estimate of 69.4% for the risk ratio and a 95% probability interval from 54.6% to 88.2%.

5. DISCUSSION

The estimation of treatment effects is receiving greater emphasis in the reporting of clinical trials [7,8], and so it is important to recognise the effect of stopping rules on estimation. Group sequential methods for designing a clinical trial allow for early termination of a trial when there is reasonable evidence that one treatment is better than another. However, by simulation, we have shown that estimates of treatment effect derived from trials using these designs are exaggerated, though the average level of bias is relatively small. More importantly the reported estimates from clinical trials that stop early, particularly if at the first or second interim analysis, lack precision, are of necessity large and may even be totally unrealistic. The reported estimates will seem unexpectedly large to the clinical reader though he may also be distracted into believing them because the associated P-value is very small (to enable stopping of the trial), and because the trial was well designed with the potential for a large number of patients to have been entered. Classical methods of bias adjustment only produce minor reductions in these estimates because they condition upon the possibility of later stopping (equivalently upon uncollected data) given a true underlying effect.

We have shown how Bayes Theorem can be applied to produce more plausible estimates of treatment effect. This approach has the particular advantage that it produces greater shrinkage of estimates of treatment effect when the trial stops early and sampling variation in the data is most important. However, note that increased accumulation of data reduces the influence of the prior adopted. Of course, the method does require the specification of prior belief and our approach for this has been reasonably simplistic. If previous trials of the therapies under consideration have been carried out, then results from these may be incorporated. Alternatively, Freedman and Speigelhalter [9] have described a method of seeking prior opinion by interviewing the clinical investigators involved in a clinical trial. Clearly, whatever method is used, the choice of prior is not unique and any prior adopted must be realistic. In particular, those produced by individuals with particular interests in the treatment under test (e.g. commercial) might be questioned. In this respect a trial report should always present the data obtained and a conventional method of inference described. In using a supplementary Bayesian approach, indication can then be made of the sensitivity of the estimates presented to the prior distribution used. How to present such results to a non-statistical audience requires careful consideration.

A useful byproduct of the Bayesian approach is that the prior distribution obtained might be used to define alternative stopping rules. Classical group sequential rules can, theoretically, have any sequence of critical values for the test statistic provided that the type I error rate is preserved at some desired level. However, there is little objectivity applied to the choice of rule beyond that it may not be desirable to allow too early stopping. Instead, the shape of the stopping boundary might be chosen to make it more consistent with the prior belief determined. This might be taken a step further so that stopping rules are based upon the posterior distribution itself: this requires further investigation.

REFERENCES

[1] Geller, N. L. and Pocock, S. J. (1987) 'Interim analyses in randomized clinical trials: Ramifications and guidelines for practitioners', Biometrics, 43, 213-224.

[2] O'Brien, P. C. and Fleming, T. R. (1979) 'A multiple testing procedure for clinical trials', Biometrics, 35, 549-556.

[3] De Mets, D. L. and Ware, J. H., (1980) 'Group sequential methods in clinical trials with a one-sided hypothesis', Biometrika, 67, 651-660.

[4] AIMS Trial Study Group, (1988) 'Effect of intravenous APSAC on mortality after acute myocardial infarction: preliminary report of a placebo-controlled clinical trial', The Lancet, i, 545-549.

[5] Chang, M. N. and O'Brien, P. C. (1986) 'Confidence intervals following group sequential tests', Controlled Clinical Trials, 7, 18-26.

[6] Whitehead, J., (1986) 'On the bias of maximum likelihood estimation following a sequential test', Biometrika, 73, 573-581.

[7] Langman, M. J. S. (1986) (editorial), 'Towards estimation and confidence limits', British Medical Journal, 292, 716

[8] (editorial), (1987) 'Report with confidence', The Lancet, i, 488.

[9] Freedman, L. S. and Spiegelhalter, D. J. (1983) 'The assessment of subjective opinion and its use in relation to stopping rules for clinical trials', The Statistician, 33, 153-160.

HELPING THE DOCTOR TO PRESCRIBE: PHILEX - A COMPUTER-BASED DECISION SUPPORT SYSTEM

J.R. Ashford
(Exeter Data Base Systems Limited)

The PHILEX System is designed to assist the medical practitioner in his role as a prescriber. A local computer with terminals on the doctor's desk provides access to two data bases, one concerned with pharmaceutical products and the second with patients and their medication. The product data base covers all drugs which may be prescribed by general medical practitioners in the United Kingdom. The System provides rapid access to information in plain language about each product and to coded data relating to a variety of attributes that are important in prescribing. Access is by product name, by indication and by pharmacological action group. The patient medication data base contains personal information about patients that is relevant to prescribing, together with details of prescriptions. A suite of computer programs helps the doctor to select appropriate medication and to write a prescription. As part of this process, checks are made upon various aspects of the prescription, including interactions with existing medication, patient idiosyncracies, dosage regime, contra-indications and precautions, and warnings are issued where appropriate. A facility is also available to record the indication for which the product was prescribed and the patient's response.

Some natural extensions of the software to enhance the 'intelligence' of the System are then discussed. These include further assistance in the selection of medication by listing products which correspond to Boolean expressions in terms of the coded attributes, of 'personalising' the selection process in the context of a particular patient and of feeding back to the prescriber information about the response to particular products in relation to particular indications accumulated within the patient medication data base.

1. INTRODUCTION

Advances in technology during recent years have led to a growing range of computer applications. Many smaller businesses and groups of professional workers have recognised that modern, low-cost micro- and mini-computers have a great potential for improving the effectiveness and efficiency of their activities. Medicine is no exception to this rule and computer systems are now being introduced on a significant scale, particularly in general medical practice.

The computer applications in general practice which have so far become established (Preece, 1983) are mainly concerned with routine administrative tasks, such as patient registration, the preparation of age-sex registers, vaccination and immunisation programmes and the control of repeat prescriptions. These should be regarded as the first, hesitant steps in a process which must inevitably penetrate more deeply into the professional activities of the doctor. The next stage is to put the computer terminal on the doctor's desk and to allow him to take direct advantage of its particular capabilities.

There is little doubt that the prescription pad, backed by the resources of the pharmaceutical industry, is one of the main weapons in the doctor's armoury. However, the growing range and potency of the available products, coupled with the steady accumulation of information about their advantages and disadvantages, presents severe problems to the doctor, who is required to match the needs of the particular patient to the characteristics of the products prescribed. Prescribing is essentially a complex data processing operation: information about pharmaceutical products must be linked with information about patients and their existing medication to produce a prescription which is optimal in relation to the patient's needs. The storage and retrieval of large quantities of information is one of the functions for which the computer is well-suited and the case for using the computer to assist with the prescribing process is very strong.

2. THE PRESCRIBING PROCESS

The prescribing process involves three distinct stages:-

(i) The assessment of the patient's signs and symptoms and any other relevant information about the patient and his state of health. This process may or may not result in a firm diagnosis but we will assume that the result is an 'indication' of the patient's current problem.

(ii) The selection of a product (or several products) in

response to the patient's indication. The aim may be to achieve a cure, but is often merely to ameliorate adverse symptoms. This process involves a consideration of the patient's characteristics, medical history, current health status and existing medication in the light of the available products. Many patients, particularly the elderly, may require several products at the same time and may receive their medication on a long-term basis. As a result, the selection of a product may involve a delicate balance between advantages and disadvantages, in a situation in which the information available about particular products is incomplete (e.g. because new information is still being accumulated and assessed by the responsible bodies).

(iii) The prescription must be specified (currently on a sheet of paper) in sufficient detail for the product to be dispensed and for any relevant instructions to be transmitted to the patient.

In the face of these tasks, the current standard prescribing procedures are far from ideal. The main problems are as follows:-

(i) The volume of information on available products is such that a digest has to be provided for the prescriber. Of the many digests available, some are at variance with others and often the presentation of information is inadequate or inappropriate. Access is inconvenient, particularly during the course of a consultation, and as a result the prescriber tends to restrict his choice to a limited repertoire of products about which he feels confident.

(ii) The introduction of new products and changes in the data about existing products means that the product information base must be updated continuously. This is difficult in the context of paper-based digests which can only be revised at infrequent intervals.

(iii) In selecting a product, the prescriber must apply a range of checks in relation to product data and to the patient's records, on product specification, on interaction with other products currently being administered, on dosage regime, on known adverse reactions (patient 'idiosyncracies') to products and/or ingredients, on precautions and on contra-indications. This may be an exacting task and the dispensing pharmacist (who in theory provides a second element of decision support) does not necessarily have the information required to confirm the doctor's choice.

(iv) The doctor may not be able to remember all the relevant detail about product availability, including formulation, strength, dosage and pack sizes, especially for those products which he uses infrequently.

(v) The doctor is required to make a separate entry in the patient's medication record for each prescription, a task which is essential if an adequate medical record is to be maintained.

(vi) Instructions given to the patient regarding administration of the product may be poorly expressed, misunderstood or omitted. While written instructions are more effective than those given verbally, there is seldom sufficient time during a consultation to produce a hand-written copy for the patient. The pharmaceutical industry is currently reviewing this problem, in relation to the issue of standard 'patient inserts', but these must inevitably be of a general nature and cannot be tailored to the needs of the particular patient.

(vii) Hand-written prescriptions may be difficult to read and are a further potential source of error.

Our aim in developing a computer-assisted prescribing system is to remove the possibility of all avoidable prescribing errors, whilst at the same time making the writing of the prescription and any associated record-keeping more efficient.

3. THE PRODUCT DATA BASE

The implementation of computer-assisted prescribing must rest on the construction and maintenance of two major data bases and on the provision of software to provide the necessary access and logic to write and check the prescription. The system described below is available commercially and is known as PHILEX ('PH'armaceutical 'I'ndustry 'LEX'icon).

The first and fundamental data base concerns the available pharmaceutical products. The PHILEX data base covers all products which may be prescribed by general medical practitioners in the United Kingdom. Information about each product is provided, updated and authenticated by the company responsible for that product: a consortium of companies is responsible for information about generic products. The information included in the data base is based on the 'data sheets' produced as a statutory requirement by the company concerned.

Responsibility for the content of the product data therefore rests within the pharmaceutical industry, which has an obvious interest in accuracy, timeliness and relevance, but is also constrained by statutory legal obligations. The data base is updated at monthly intervals.

A standard set of information is provided for each product:-

(i) An identifier, comprising name, qualifier (e.g. 'forte', 'paediatric'), formulation and strength.

(ii) A summary in the English language of the main attributes of the product. This summary is derived from the corresponding 'data sheet' and is presented in a standardised format, usually within the compass of a single computer screen. An example is given as Appendix I.

(iii) A coded summary of various characteristics of the product relevant to the prescribing process. The codes for each attribute are standardised by means of a corresponding dictionary. The codes can be displayed in decoded form for inspection by the prescriber but their main function is to provide relevant data concerning the product for the prescribing software. A list of the attributes is given in Appendix II.

(iv) The clinically significant interactions of the product with each of the other products belonging to the data base.

In addition to the product information itself, the data base also includes a series of indexes designed to give rapid access to the products with defined characteristics, including indication and pharmacological action group. For example, selection by indication will produce a list of products for which that particular indication is approved. The data base also includes pointers which link all proprietary products corresponding to any defined generic product.

4. THE PATIENT DATA BASE

The second major data base concerns the patient and his medication. Before the first prescription is issued, the doctor (or, more usually his receptionist) is required to set up a simple patient record containing name and other personal identification, together with personal characteristics relevant to medication, including sex, date of birth, idiosyncracies, medical condition and overdose history. This forms the kernel of the patient medication record.

Each prescription is entered through the computer terminal

keyboard using an interactive program designed to minimise the number of key depressions. As far as possible, items are entered automatically from the product or patient data bases. During the entry process, the following checks are made and, where necessary, warnings are issued:-

(i) interactions with other current medication;

(ii) 'doubling' effects (when a new product with the same pharmacological action group as a current product is prescribed);

(iii) patient idiosyncrasy in relation to any ingredient;

(iv) dosage regime;

(v) contra-indications and warnings.

The computational powers of the computer are also used to assist in the specification of the prescription, for example, by calculating the number of tablets corresponding to a given number of days of supply on the basis of dose level and frequency. A facility is also available for the control of repeat prescriptions The completed prescription is printed on standard stationery using a printer attached to the terminal, together with selected patient instructions on a 'tear-off' section. As an aid to rapid prescribing, the System allows the doctor to set up a personal prescribing 'repertoire' containing his most commonly-used prescriptions, from which a selection can be made with the minimum number of key depressions.

If a check is violated, the program allows the doctor to respond with the least possible inconvenience (e.g. by giving access to the product data base to allow another product to be selected). However, the doctor is free to ignore any warning and to continue with the prescribing process if so desired.

As part of the prescription-writing process, a facility is provided for the doctor to enter the relevant indication. This is done using the same dictionary as is used for the coding of indications in the product data base and permits the analysis of the medication records in terms of morbidity on an unambiguous basis A facility is also provided to review each prescription in terms of effectiveness in treating the indication and also in terms of side-effects. As the System is used, a data base is accumulated for each patient showing personal information and details of each prescription, together with the associated indication and response. This data base grows as the System is used and offers the possibility of providing further assistance in the prescribing process.

5. TOWARDS A MORE 'EXPERT' SYSTEM

The facilities described above are all commercially available and are being increasingly widely used within general practice. However, they can be regarded as merely a first step towards an expert system to assist in the prescribing process. The next logical steps are as follows:-

(i) To provide access to lists of products on the basis of any defined set of coded attributes.

The existing facilities provide access on the basis of indication or pharmacological action group only. A natural extension, which would be of considerable potential value in the selection of an appropriate product, is to provide access on the basis of a Boolean function of any set of the coded attributes. For example, a list of products for treating asthma which are not contra-indicated by pregnancy but may be taken by inhalation could well be useful to a prescriber.

(ii) To 'personalise' access to the product data base in the context of a particular patient.

For prescribing purposes, access to the date base is made after the identity of the patient has been established. This offers the possibility of qualifying all product information derived from the data base in terms of the attributes and medication record of that patient. Thus, access in terms of indication would generate a list of products recommended for that indication, but qualified in the light of the circumstances of the particular patient. For example, the doctor could avoid selecting a particular product, only to be forced to choose an alternative during the course of writing the prescription if an interaction with existing medication were to be detected at that stage.

(iii) To take account of information accumulated in the patient medication record.

The medication record for an individual patient contains potentially useful information about the response of that patient to previous medication prescribed for a specified indication. This information should be made available to the doctor when he is writing a further prescription, particularly if this is in relation to the same indication or product.

(iv) To take account of information accumulated in the patient medication data base about groups of patients.

The latter data base contains potentially useful information about groups of patients, for example about the response of a given class of patients to a range of products prescribed to treat a defined condition. The larger the data base, the more useful would be the information which might be accumulated in this way, but for a group practice with, say, 10,000 patients, a significant body of knowledge about the more common causes of morbidity or about the products more commonly prescribed might be generated over a period of one or two years. Immediate access to information of this type would only be possible as a result of periodic summaries of the data base carried out 'off-line'. The most appropriate form of summarisation cannot be determined without a formal evaluation of alternatives. On general grounds, it is clear that an analysis of all prescriptions involving a particular product and of all prescriptions relating to a given indication must form the basis of an effective system. The summarisation of such data in a form which might be useful for decision support must involve a statistical approach to the interpretation of comparative data. The value of an internally-generated data base of this kind of course reflects the past practice of the prescribers and is limited in the context of new products. The pooling of many data bases of this type would serve to produce information of wider application, but at the expense of the blurring of definitions used in recording indications and responses.

6. TECHNOLOGY

The PHILEX System was originally designed to run on a micro- or mini-computer with 640 KB core and 'hard disk' storage of up to 40 MB. With the advent of cheaper mass storage media such as the compact disk (CD), which allows much greater volumes of data to be accessed at comparable speed, the content of the product data base is being reviewed and it is envisaged that the existing English language summaries will be supplemented by much more detailed textual and graphical information.

The greater reliability of telecommunication equipment offers the practical possibility of linking together patient medication data bases from many practices. This will make possible for the first time the accumulation of a timely and representative body of quantitative knowledge about the effectiveness and disadvantages of particular products with obvious advantages for the evaluation of both new and well-established products. Such information may be fed back to the doctor to improve the quality of prescribing generally.

Although technical issues are important, the main limitation to the effective use of systems of this kind is cultural. The prescriber must be prepared to accept that his professional skills can be enhanced by the disciplined use of an expert system which should free him of more mundane responsibilities to concentrate upon the more challenging and serious issues. In the context of prescribing in the United Kingdom, there is little doubt that iatrogenic disease caused by avoidable prescribing errors is a serious problem which in itself is sufficient to justify the introduction of systems such as PHILEX on a general basis.

7. ACKNOWLEDGEMENTS

The author is obliged to Dr. John Preece, whose ideas and experience of general practice have had a fundamental influence on the development of the PHILEX System, and to Mr. C.N. Whitt and Mrs. M.A. Ramsden for valuable discussions and advice.

8. REFERENCE

Preece, J.F. (1983) The Use of Computers in General Practice. Library of General Practice, No. 5. Edinburgh: Churchill Livingstone.

APPENDIX I

Example of Product Information in Plain Language

```
DIUREXAN                    POM                          E MERCK LTD 0420 640

DIUREXAN TABLETS            20MG XIPAMIDE        ROUND/ SCORED/ WHITE/ MARKED
USES:    HYPERTENSION/ OEDEMA
ACTION: DIURETIC/ANTIHYPERTENSIVE/ GENTLE ONSET OF ACTION/ GRADUAL PROLONGED
        EFFECT/ DIURETIC ACTIVITY LASTS UP TO 12 HOURS/ ANTIHYPERTENSIVE EFFECT
        EVIDENT FOR 24 HOURS OR MORE
DOSAGE: SINGLE EARLY MORNING DOSE/ HYPERTENSION 1-2 TABLETS DAILY/
        OEDEMA INITIAL DOSE 2 TABLETS DAILY/DECREASE TO 1 WHEN CONTROL ADEQUATE
        INCREASE TO 4 IN RESISTANT CASES/ NOT RECOMMENDED FOR CHILDREN
CONTRA-INDICATIONS: SEVERE ELECTROLYTE DEFICIENCY/ PRECOMATOSE STATES ASSOCIATE
                    WITH LIVER CIRRHOSIS/ SEVERE RENAL INSUFFICIENCY
PRECAUTIONS:  PREGNANCY/ LONG TERM THERAPY MAY INDUCE HYPOKALAEMIA
              HYPERURICAEMIA OR CHANGED GLUCOSE METABOLISM MAY OCCUR IN PRE-
              DISPOSED PATIENTS/ ACUTE RETENTION MAY OCCUR IN PATIENTS WITH
              PROSTATIC HYPERTROPHY
SIDE EFFECTS: SLIGHT GI DISTURBANCE AND MILD DIZZINESS OCCASIONALLY REPORTED
OVERDOSAGE:   MAINTAIN BLOOD PRESSURE/ RESTORE BLOOD VOLUME AND ELECTROLYTE
              BALANCE
STORAGE:      PROTECT FROM HEAT AND MOISTURE
INTERACTIONS: DOSAGE OF HYPOTENSIVE DRUGS CARDIAC GLYCOSIDES
              HYPOGLYCAEMIC AGENTS OR INSULIN MAY NEED ADJUSTING

Press ↵ to continue                              Date of last edit 24/09/1986
```

APPENDIX II

Coded Attributes in Product Data Base

Indications (Uses)
Action Groups
Body Systems
Ingredients
Co-idiosyncrasy Action Groups and Ingredients
Prescribing Category
Contra-Indications
Precautions
Warnings
Dosage Information
Mandatory Instructions
Pack Information

ASSESSING THE ROLE OF DIET IN CANCER EPIDEMIOLOGY IN SINGAPORE

S.W. Duffy
(MRC Biostatistics Unit, Cambridge)

and

H.P. Lee and L. Gourley
(Department of Community, Occupational and Family Medicine, National University of Singapore)

ABSTRACT

Recent work on diet and cancer in Singapore provides an excellent example of the process of thought linking descriptive and analytic epidemiology. Incidence rates of different cancers have been changing dramatically in Singapore in recent years. Rates of cancers of the oesophagus and stomach have been falling, while lung, colon, rectum and female breast cancer rates have been increasing. The changes suggest a degree of westernisation. There is contemporaneous evidence of a marked change in diet, with the increasing affluence of the country. Together, these results suggest a potential role of diet in disease aetiology and indicate a need for projects aimed at directly assessing the association between diet and cancers of individual sites. Case control studies of diet and colorectal, breast and nasopharyngeal cancers are at various stages of execution. Analytic strategies and preliminary results are described.

1. INTRODUCTION

This paper has minimal formal mathematical content, but it illustrates the convergence of disciplines, including medical statistics, upon the problems of chronic diseases epidemiology. The subject matter, cancer epidemiology in Singapore, gives a good example of the process involved. The one quantitative definition the reader should know is that of relative risk. The risk of disease x for group A relative to group B is

$$\frac{\text{Probability of disease x for those in group A}}{\text{Probability of disease x for those in group B}}$$

Singapore is an island at the southern tip of Peninsular Malaysia. It measures 42 kilometres from east to west and 23 kilometres from north to south. It is a city state of 2.4 million inhabitants at the 1980 census. The climate is hot and wet.

There are three main ethnic groups, Chinese (77% of the population), Malay (15%) and Indian (6%). The work reported on here deals with the majority Chinese population.

The Singapore Cancer Registry was founded in 1967 [8]. It has registered cancer cases since 1st January 1968. The medical and social infrastructure of Singapore is particularly suitable for comprehensive registration. Between 1968 and 1983, approximately 60,000 cancer cases were registered, of which 48,000 were malignancies in permanent residents of Singapore. Only 5% of registrations were from death certificate only, indicating thorough registration.

2. TRENDS IN CANCER INCIDENCE

Table 1 shows incidence rates of major cancers in the 5-year periods 1968-72, 1973-77 and 1978-82, standardised to the approximate age structure of the world population [9]. Incidence rates are customarily analysed by log-linear modelling [1], producing relative risk estimates, trend estimates, and tests of significance of these. This analysis indicated that there were significant trends of increasing risk with time for male and female lung, colon and rectum cancers and female breast cancer. Significant trends of decreasing risk were noted for male and female stomach and oesophageal cancers.
Further analysis indicated that birth cohort effects were more effective than temporal effects for describing changes in breast and lung cancer incidence [4,5]. A birth cohort effect can be thought of as an interaction between age and period, ie the difference in incidence between two age groups at period a is not the same as that difference at period b. In this case, year of birth is a better predictor of risk than age. Risks by cohort are shown for male lung cancer and female breast cancer, relative to the cohort with mid-point 1928, in Table 2. Note that for breast cancer, risk is low for the oldest cohort and generally steadily increases with each successive cohort. The relative risk for those born after 1950 is particularly high. These suggest changes in lifestyle or environment which affect risk, but do not apply to people of all ages at a given time. For breast cancer, one such possibility is a change in diet, but changes in reproductive habits could be equally responsible [5].

The temporal trends were noted some years ago [8]. In perhaps over-simplistic terms, the trends represent a change

Table 1 CANCER INCIDENCE[1] IN SINGAPORE 1968-82

(a) Males

Site	Rates (% of 68-72) for periods 1968-72	1973-77	1978-82
Lung	57.0(100)	66.2(116)	73.3(129)
Stomach	44.9(100)	42.1(94)	37.3(83)
Liver	33.9(100)	31.1(92)	31.6(93)
Nasopharynx	19.0(100)	19.9(105)	18.1(95)
Oesophagus	20.0(100)	17.4(87)	13.5(68)
Colon	12.1(100)	14.0(116)	16.4(136)
Rectum	10.2(100	13.7(134)	14.6(143)

(b) Females

Site	Rates (% of 67-72) for calendar period 1968-72	1973-77	1978-82
Breast	19.5(100)	22.4(115)	27.1(139)
Lung	17.3(100)	19.9(115)	22.7(131)
Cervix U.	18.8(100)	18.3(97)	16.9(92)
Stomach	18.4(100)	17.8(97)	15.3(83)
Colon	9.6(100)	12.9(134)	15.9(166)
Rectum	7.1(100)	8.2(115)	10.6(149)
Liver	8.2(100)	7.4(90)	7.3(89)

[1] Rates per 100,000 person-years for Chinese residents, age - standardised to the world population

Table 2 EXAMPLES OF COHORT EFFECTS

Relative risk by year of birth, relative to 1928 birth cohort, for male lung and female breast cancers

Cohort mid-point or	Sex and Site Male Lung	Female Breast
1950 onwards	0.74	3.47
1948	1.07	2.50
1943	0.80	2.29
1938	1.07	1.89
1933	0.97	1.18
1928	1.00	1.00
1923	0.92	0.83
1918	0.85	0.83
1913	0.80	0.74
1908	0.74	0.65
1903	0.60	0.66
1898	0.50	0.55
Pre-1897	0.37	0.40

from the traditional "Chinese" pattern of malignancy to that prevailing in the West. The recent increase in material affluence in Singapore, and the temporal changes in rates of stomach, colon, rectum and breast cancers suggested a search for dietary agents might be worth pursuing. Accordingly, the International Agency for Research on Cancer set up a Diet Study Group in the National University of Singapore in 1984.

3. DIETARY SURVEYS

One of the first studies by the Diet Study Group was an investigation of changes in food availability in Singapore since 1961 [6]. Availability of almost all foods was greater in the period 1976-80 than in 1961-65, but the difference was particularly marked for meat, fruit and eggs. The availability of meat, one of the more expensive foods, increased from 69g per capita per day in 1961-65 to 163g per capita per day in 1976-80, an increase of 136%.

A survey of foods purchased for home consumption in 40 households confirmed the finding that present-day consumption is considerably higher than two decades ago [2]. Further, when the subjects were categorised as of high or low affluence, using housing status to measure affluence, distinctly higher intakes were noted for the "high affluence" groups, particularly for more expensive items such as red meat and fruit (see Table 3). Thus increased affluence has conceivably made a considerable difference to the diet of the population. A three-day food diary survey of 98 individuals yielded more detailed information on individual dietary intakes (Gourley, personal communication). Mean fat intake among males under 40 years was 64g/day (95% data range 34-122g/day) and among females aged under 40 the mean intake was 46g/day (95% range 21-103). For dietary fibre intakes, the averages were both roughly 13g/day with 95% ranges of about 5-25g/day.

All these findings indicate consumption levels lower than those in the west but much higher than in Singapore 20 years ago. They also indicate a wide extent of variation (ie there are people still having the more frugal intakes common in the past). This is understandable in a society which has undergone a large economic and social transition. Thus, in direct study of diet and disease the high and low consumption groups can be well-represented, yielding a good potential for distinguishing between high and low risk groups.

4. DIRECT STUDY OF DIET AND DISEASE

The most common tool in analytic epidemiology is the case-

Table 3 SURVEY OF FOODS PURCHASED:

Median (Inter-quartile range) in g/capita/week of food groups, by housing type (1="high affluence", 2= "low affluence")

Food Group	Type 1	Type 2	Both	p-value
Red Meat	775 (436,996)	286 (249,445)	437 (276,750)	0.001
Poultry	388 (351,856)	250 (21,461)	353 (214,583)	0.002
Fish	608 (385,687)	442 (378,842)	600 (386,746)	0.95
Green veg.	707 (465,1154)	679 (462,854)	679 (473,880)	0.8
Other veg.	870 (460,1188)	438 (317,756)	654 (383,918)	0.04
Fruit	1793 (567,2542)	710 (434,889)	801 (542,1855)	0.007
No. households	14	17	31	

NB Excludes 9 households who ate in less than half the time

control study, in which the histories of patients with a given disease are compared with those of subjects without the disease (the controls). The above results suggested that case-control studies of diet and colorectal cancer and diet and breast cancer might be fruitful. A hospital-based case-control study of colorectal cancer has been completed and analysis thereof is at an advanced stage. The questionnaire was designed using information from the surveys described in Section 3. Preliminary results indicate a relative risk of 0.50 to be associated with high consumption of cruciferous vegetables, and a relative risk of 1.77 in association with a high meat-to-vegetable consumption ratio. These add to and further quantify the body of evidence for these effects already in the literature [3,7].

Recruitment to a case-control study of breast cancer and diet is almost complete. A study of diet and nasopharyngeal cancer is planned.

5. DISCUSSION

It is hoped that the foregoing has provided an illustration of the steps in the progression from descriptive to analytic epidemiology. We start with descriptive epidemiology, the study of rates of disease in the community, which requires good quality disease registration and vital statistics. This in turn generates hypotheses about the agents responsible for spatial or temporal disease patterns. Study of the potential casual agents (in this case the dietary surveys) is not indispensable, but can be a valuable intermediate step. It is worthwhile to check that the potential agents are changing contemporaneously with the disease rates and in a manner compatible with the hypotheses generated. It also has the beneficial effect of "testing the water", giving the researchers information about which research strategies are suitable in the field. In the present case, this step was particularly valuable in that it provided information about ranges of intake, suggesting that there was sufficient variability to distinguish high- and low-risk groups. The final stage is the direct assessment of associations between disease and potential predisposing or protective agents. If the earlier work has been thorough, the researchers can be confident of useful information resulting from the final stage. This seems to be borne out by the findings of the case-control study of colorectal cancer and diet.

ACKNOWLEDGEMENTS

We thank the International Agency for Research on Cancer for financial support. For assistance in the various studies described we are grateful to N. E. Day of the MRC Biostatistics

Unit, Cambridge, K. Shanmugaratnam of the Singapore Cancer Registry, J. Lee and C. Y. Tye of the Department of Community, Occupational and Family Medicine, National University of Singapore, S. W. Goh of the Computer Centre, National University of Singapore and J. Estève of the International Agency for Research on Cancer.

REFERENCES

[1] Breslow, N. E. and Day, N. E. (1987) "Statistical Methods in Cancer Research Volume II - The Design and Analysis of Cohort Studies", International Agency for Research on Cancer, Lyon.

[2] Gourley, L., Duffy, S. W., Lee, H. P., Walker A. M. and Day, N. E. (1988) "A Survey of Household Food Purchases and Dietary Habits in Relation to Affluence among Singapore Chinese.". European Journal of Clinical Nutrition, 42, 333-343.

[3] La Vecchia, C., Negri, E., Decarli, A., D'Avanzo, B., Gallotti, L., Gentile, A. and Franceschi, S. (1988) "A Case-control Study of Diet and Colo-rectal Cancer in Northern Italy". International Journal of Cancer, 412, 492-498.

[4] Lee, H. P., Day, N. E. and Shanmugaratnam, K. (1988) "Trends in Cancer Incidence in Singapore, 1968-1982". International Agency for Research on Cancer, Lyon.

[5] Lee, H. P., Duffy, S. W., Day, N. E. and Shanmugaratnam, K. (1988) "Recent Trends in Cancer Incidence among Singapore Chinese". International Journal of Cancer, 42, 159-166.

[6] Lee, H. P. and Gourley, L. (1986) "Food Availability in Singapore, 1961-1983". Implications for Health Research, Food and Nutrition Bulletin of the United Nations University, 8, 50-54.

[7] Manousos, O., Day, N. E., Trichopoulos, D., Gerovassilis, F., Tzonou, A. and Polychronopoulou, A. (1983) "Diet and Colorectal Cancer: A Case-control Study in Greece". International Journal of Cancer, 32, 1-5.

[8] Shanmugaratnam, K., Lee, H. P. and Day, N. E. (1983) "Cancer Incidence in Singapore, 1968-77". International Agency for Research on Cancer, Lyon.

[9] Waterhouse, J., Muir, C., Shanmugaratnam, K. and Powell, J. (eds). (1982) "Cancer Incidence in Five Continents, Volume IV". International Agency for Research on Cancer, Lyon.

DISCRIMINANT ANALYSIS APPLIED TO AN ORTHOPAEDIC PROBLEM

C. C. Patterson, W. G. Kernohan and R. A. B. Mollan
(The Queen's University of Belfast, Belfast)

ABSTRACT

Screening tests for orthopaedic disorders often involve the subjective perception of subtle signs from the patient's joints. For example in Barlow's test for congenital dislocation of the hip, the examiner performs a gentle manoeuvre of the neonatal hip while feeling for abnormal "clunks" or "clicks". A system, based on miniature accelerometers, has been developed to assist with the interpretation of Barlow's test. Over six hundred transient signals from more than three hundred hips have been recorded.

Variables characterising the signals were derived using a dual microprocessor arrangement and these were subsequently transferred to a mainframe computer. Discriminant analysis using the classical linear discriminant function method and a kernel density estimation method was employed to determine how successfully features of the recorded signals could differentiate between clinically defined groups. The discriminatory ability of the methods and the reliability of their allocation probabilities are compared.

An allocation rule has been implemented in an Amstrad P.C. and a commercial package for early diagnosis of hip dislocation in the neonate has been manufactured.

1. INTRODUCTION

Congenital dislocation of the hip (CDH) is a condition of the newborn or young infant in which the head of the femur does not correctly locate in the acetabulum. The trained orthopaedic surgeon can detect instability of the hip at birth. However, some cases are not detectable and only become clinically apparent in the first few years of life. Often the condition is diagnosed when the child presents walking with a limp. If detected early, treatment with a nappy splint is very successful and has minimal complications. However, late detection typically results in the need for traction, operation and a prolonged period in plaster, with far from satisfactory results. Further operations may be necessary, and often the child continues to walk with a limp and suffers from osteoarthritis in later life.

The condition shows interesting epidemiological features, many of which have been known for some time. In Table 1 obstetric and perinatal data recorded in the Northern Ireland Child Health System for 187 cases of CDH born in the period 1983-85 are compared with corresponding data on all Northern Ireland births in the same period. The overall incidence rate was 2.29 per 1,000 live births but there was an eight fold excess in girls compared with boys. Some seasonal variation was evident with higher incidence in the autumn and winter months. There was a very obvious excess of cases among breech presentations. Also there was a suggestion that CDH was associated with a prolonged labour, and this could not be explained by breech presentations having a longer labour. Babies with CDH were slightly more mature and their mothers were slightly older. Previous studies have shown primigravida mothers to be at especially high risk of having children with CDH, but this was not evident in Northern Ireland data. There were no social class differences in CDH incidence. Seventy-nine (42%) of the 187 cases were diagnosed late (i.e. when the child was aged six months or more).

The desirability of early detection has resulted in the development of screening procedures. In the Ortolani and Barlow stress tests [1] the infant's hips are carefully manipulated under light pressure. A dislocatable hip will produce a characteristic *clunk* which the experienced examiner will hear or feel. However about 10% of newborn babies produce a *click* which the untrained examiner may find difficult to distinguish from the clunk of the unstable hip.

These screening procedures are in widespread use, but their introduction has not always reduced the incidence of late detection of CDH [9]. In contrast, others have reported that they are able to detect most cases of CDH at birth [3]. Part of the explanation for this apparent discrepancy almost certainly lies in the level of experience of the individual who performs the screening tests.

With this in mind we have attempted to measure the vibration emissions from the neonatal hip obtained during the screening procedure and to use variables derived from the resulting signals to emulate the experienced examiner.

		CDH cases (n=187)	All births (N=81,598)	Rate per 1,000 livebirths
Sex	Male	21	42,047	0.50
	Female	166	39,546	4.20
	Not known	-	5	-
Month of Birth	Dec-Feb	50	19,294	2.59
	Mar-May	43	21,090	2.04
	Jun-Aug	42	20,931	2.01
	Sep-Nov	52	20,278	2.56
	Not known	-	5	-
Previous Pregnancies	0	33	14,216	2.32
	1	63	21,643	2.91
	2	27	14,634	1.85
	≥ 3	38	19,147	1.98
	Not known	26	11,958	-
Presentation	Normal	132	64,450	2.05
	Breech	17	1,368	12.43
	Section	17	7,465	2.28
	Other/not known	21	8,315	-
Duration of Labour	< 6 hours	107	49,262	2.17
	6-11 hours	56	24,687	2.27
	≥ 12 hours	15	4,133	3.63
	Not known	9	3,516	-
Social Class	I or II	41	16,970	2.42
	III	91	34,555	2.63
	IV or V	38	14,892	2.55
	Other/not known	17	15,181	-
Birthweight	Mean ± SD (g)	3431 ± 501	3389 ± 558	
Gestation	Mean ± SD (wk)	39.4 ± 1.3	39.1 ± 1.8	
Mother's Age	Mean ± SD (yr)	28.5 ± 5.5	27.6 ± 5.6	

Source: N. Ireland Child Health Record System

Table 1 Obstetric and perinatal data for cases of congenital hip dislocation and all live births in N. Ireland 1983-85.

2. MATERIAL

We used three small accelerometers (Bruel & Kjaer type 4344) to detect vibrations from neonatal hip joints as they were being carefully manipulated. Two of these accelerometers were taped to the skin in the region of the anterior iliac crests. It was possible to attach them by cutting a cruciate hole in the adhesive tape and passing the barrel of the sensor through the hole and securing both the base and cable to the skin. Another accelerometer was attached to a foam plate on which the baby lay during testing. This sensor was in contact with the upper sacral skin.

The Ortolani and Barlow tests were carried out by a skilled operator. Episodes of vibration which occurred during testing were amplified (Bruel & Kjaer type 2635) and recorded on a four channel frequency modulated tape deck (Bruel & Kjaer type 7003). A footswitch was used to indicate the position of palpable events.

The signals were then replayed into a multichannel ink-jet recorder (Elema-Schonander Mingograf 34). Thus valid vibration episodes could be identified for further analysis by their simultaneous appearance on replay on at least two accelerometer channels, one of which was the hip being examined. The foot-switch channel revealed palpable episodes from the recording and this was used in identification. Little regard was paid to relative amplitude across the three channels since this depended on attachment quality and tissue medium through which the vibration travelled. In the case of Ortolani's test, where both hips are abducted together and a vibration episode was detected but not palpated then the small phase lead of the accelerometer channel nearest to the joint producing the signal was used to indicate the channel for further analysis. In addition, hip vibration could be recognised and distinguished from background noise and from noise produced when the baby was released from the examiner's hands. When a valid episode was detected and the channel identified in this way, it was replayed, often several times, into a narrow band spectrum analyser (Bruel & Kjaer type 2031) and transferred via a laboratory interface (IEEE-488) to a microcomputer (Apple II).

A signal analysis program was written to allow time windowing and to compute a series of variables used to characterise the vibration event. Most of the variables were obtained from consideration of the signal in the time domain, but two variables were obtained from consideration of the signal in the frequency domain after a Fourier transform had been applied by the spectrum analyser. The variables calculated for each vibration episode were:-

peak positive acceleration (m/s^2),

peak negative acceleration (m/s^2),

acceleration range (m/s^2),

pulse area (m/s),

root mean square (RMS) acceleration (m/s^2),

positive decay factor,

negative decay factor,

peak frequency (Hz)

and level of the peak frequency (dB relative to 1μV).

To facilitate transfer of information from the Apple microcomputer to a mainframe computer for statistical analysis, a computer file was written for each event to record these variables together with sampling frequency, analogue to digital converter range, tape recorder playback speed and amplifier setting. The file also contained the vibration event itself stored as a series of values.

Between August 1981 and July 1982 the above method which has come to be known as *vibration arthrometry* was used to detect vibration events during the examination of infant hips. The children were mainly examined at the Royal Maternity Hospital but there were referrals from other Belfast maternity units. During routine clinical testing at five days of age by the paediatric staff attached to the units, neonates who were found to have a click or any palpable vibration in either hip were referred for vibration *arthrometry*. On later review children were again assessed by the same method. The children were divided into five clinical groups as shown in Table 2.

Fifty-three *normal* children were screened as a control group and were tested by the paediatrician and the authors but no abnormality was detected. To establish that these children did not subsequently develop CDH they were clinically reviewed. Twenty-two were seen until 4.5 years of age, 12 were seen between 1 and 3 years and one at six months. Eight were cleared by their general practitioner and nine mothers responded favourably to a questionnaire when the child was aged 4. There was one death.

Clinical group	Result of neonatal examination	Diagnosis	Infants	Infants with signals	Hips with Signals	Vibration episodes
Normal	Normal	Normal	53	19	26	36
Safe click	Click	Normal	201	156	289	434
CDH click	Click	CDH	16	15	30	49
Unstable	Clunk	Early CDH	14	10	18	48
Late clunk	-	Late CDH	22	13	17	62
All groups			306	213	380	629

Table 2 Definition of clinical groups and details of recorded vibration episodes.

In 201 cases a vibration was felt on examination but no clinical instability was detected and no treatment was necessary throughout. Of these, 82 were reviewed until 4 years of age and 68 between 1 and 2 years. Twelve were cleared by their GP and 36 responded favourably to the questionnaire when the child was aged 4. Three could not be traced. These cases form the *safe click* group.

In 16 cases vibration was felt on examination. Although no instability was detected at birth these children subsequently developed an abnormality at an average age of 25 weeks. They are described as the *CDH click* group.

The *unstable* group were examined as neonates and found to have a clinical abnormality. Nearly all of the 14 children in this group were subsequently treated for CDH.

Finally 22 children with a late dislocation (the *late CDH* group) were screened by vibration arthrometry at the time of closed reduction in the operating theatre.

3. METHODS

Two methods of discriminant analysis suitable for continuous variables were used and the findings obtained from the methods compared. Of particular interest are the allocation probabilities since, if shown to be trustworthy [7], these could be supplied to the clinician to help make appropriate decisions about patient management.

Classical linear discriminant analysis [8] requires assumptions of multivariate normality and equality of variance/covariance matrices if allocation probabilities are to be relied upon. A stepwise approach to variable selection was used as implemented in BMDP program P7M [7].

Discriminant analysis based on kernel density estimation [5] requires no such assumptions. In the univariate case the density function, $f(x)$, for any given group is estimated from the sample, $x_1, x_2, \ldots, x_n$ as

$$\hat{f}(x) = \frac{1}{n\,h} \sum_{i=1}^{n} k\left(\frac{x - x_i}{h}\right) \qquad (3.1)$$

where $k(.)$ is the kernel function

and h determines the amount of smoothing.

In the univariate normal situation with a Gaussian kernel function, Fryer [4] describes how h may be chosen for a given value of n to minimise an error criterion. A more general approach to choosing a value for h based on a modified maximum likelihood argument has been suggested [6].

The kernel method may be readily extended to the multivariate case. If $\underline{x}_i' = (x_{1i}, x_{2i}, \ldots, x_{pi})$ for observation i $(i=1,\ldots,n)$ then estimate $f(\underline{x})$ by

$$\hat{f}(\underline{x}) = \frac{1}{n\,h_1 \ldots h_p} \sum_{i=1}^{n} K\left(\frac{x_1 - x_{1i}}{h_1}, \frac{x_2 - x_{2i}}{h_2}, \ldots, \frac{x_p - x_{pi}}{h_p}\right) \qquad (3.2)$$

The multivariate kernel, $K(.)$, may be defined as a product of p univariate kernels

$$K\,(.) = \prod_{v=1}^{p} k\left(\frac{x_v - x_{vi}}{h_v}\right) \qquad v = 1,\ldots,p \qquad (3.3)$$

Some simplification is achieved by setting $h_1 = h_2 = \ldots h_p = h$. The modified likelihood approach may then be used to obtain the value for h which maximises

$$\prod_{j=1}^{n} \frac{1}{(n-1)h^{p}} \sum_{\substack{i=1 \\ i \neq j}}^{n} K \left\{ \frac{x_1 - x_{1i}}{h}, \frac{x_2 - x_{2i}}{h}, \ldots, \frac{x_p - x_{pi}}{h} \right\} \quad (3.4)$$

subject to the constraint $h > 0$. The NAG library routine E04JAF was used to perform this maximisation. Variables were standardised in preparation for kernel density estimation by subtracting the group mean and dividing by the group standard deviation.

For any given $\underline{x}$, a density estimate was obtained for each group and an allocation rule derived by appropriate weighting of the estimate by the prior probability for the group. In assessing the success of the method, since no independent test set was available, a leaving-one-out approach was adopted. Each case was allocated on the basis of density estimates derived only from the remaining cases.

No variable selection algorithm was incorporated in the program.

4. RESULTS

Table 2 also shows the number of children in each group whose vibration arthrometry was positive (i.e. at least one signal was recorded). In none of the groups was all cases positive on vibration arthrometry. Often both hips provided signals. Also a given hip could be positive under repeated testing so that more than one episode was recorded. A total of 629 vibration episodes was obtained.

Hips with multiple vibration episodes were used to examine the reproducibility of signal characteristics. Coefficients of variation for signal to signal variability were calculated for each of 48 hips in the safe click group using a total of 122 vibration episodes recorded in the first week of life. For each variable (with the exception of dB at peak which is measured on a logarithmic scale) the average coefficient of variation over the 48 hips was of the order of 30-40%, indicating that reproducibility of signal characteristics was poor. Values of the variables derived from each vibration episode for a given hip were averaged before further analysis.

Typical examples of vibration episodes from each group are shown in Figure 1, which indicates some subtle differences.

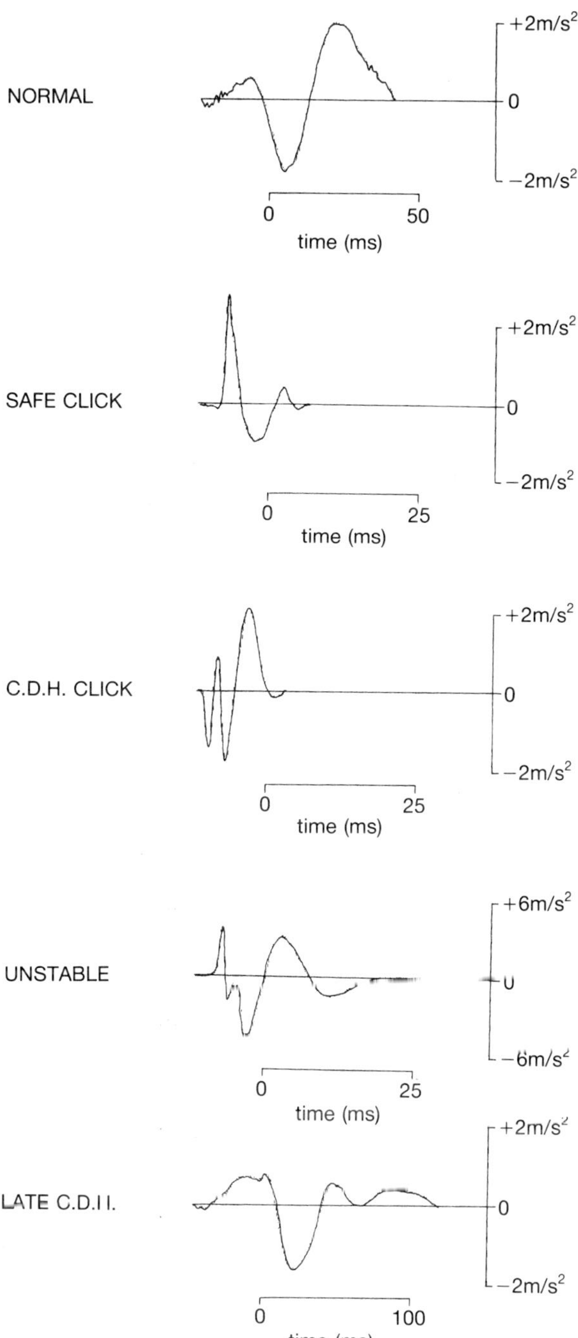

Fig. 1 Typical examples of signals considered in the time domain for each of five clinically defined groups.

Noting the differences in scale, careful scrutiny reveals, for example, that the safe click trace contains higher frequencies and has a much lower pulse area than the unstable trace.

Preliminary analysis showed that signal characteristics were correlated with the age of the infant. As the primary aim was to emulate the clinical observer performing the screening test in the period shortly after birth, the analyses described in this paper are restricted to measurements made on infants aged 7 days or less. This restriction resulted in signals being available from 16 normal hips, 133 safe clicks, 7 CDH clicks, 5 unstable hips and 0 late CDH hips.

Initial analysis also confirmed the clinical impression that it is not possible to distinguish CDH clicks from safe clicks. Rather than combining these two groups, the small CDH click group was set aside to see how it would be allocated by a discrimination rule which attempted to distinguish between normal hips, safe clicks and unstable hips. This three group discrimination approach is in keeping with current clinical practice. Infants whose hips are judged to be normal require no follow-up, infants for whom clicks are felt are routinely reviewed while infants whose hips are thought to be unstable are referred for an orthopaedic opinion.

For a number of signals the decay factors could not be calculated. Also maximum and minimum acceleration correlated very highly with acceleration range. These variables were therefore not considered further. Table 3 shows a comparison of the rest of the variables in the three remaining clinical groups. As many of the variables exhibited positive skew they were log-transformed before analysis of variance or discriminant analysis was performed.

Stepwise linear discriminant analysis was used first to determine how successfully these variables in combination could distinguish between the three groups. Peak frequency, pulse area and RMS acceleration were selected in that order, and the allocation of the 154 cases resulting from the discriminant functions is noted in Table 4(a). Of course the discriminant functions may work less well than is indicated by this table because an independent test set should be used to assess performance. However the use of the leaving-one-out (jackknife) method for allocation did not result in any deterioration in performance.

Variable	Normal (n=16)	Safe click (n=133)	Unstable (n=5)	Significance
Acceleration range (m/s^2)	3.53 ± 1.38	4.80 ± 3.63	6.87 ± 4.05	P>0.10 +
Pulse area (m/s)	0.07 ± 0.05	0.12 ± 0.12	0.81 ± 0.38	P<0.005 +
RMS acceleration (m/s^2)	1.54 ± 0.68	1.51 ± 0.89	3.90 ± 0.94	P<0.005 +
Peak frequency (Hz)	29.3 ± 32.6	118.3 ± 74.3	31.3 ± 24.1	P<0.001 +
Decibels at peak (dB)	86.4 ± 6.8	81.2 ± 7.4	88.8 ± 6.3	P<0.005

+ Log-transformed before analysis of variance.

Table 3 Comparison between clinical groups of variables derived from vibration episodes (Mean ± SD).

The kernel density method was applied using data for all five variables in Table 3. The values obtained for the smoothing parameter, h, for the three groups were 0.561, 0.359 and 0.959 for the normal, safe click and unstable groups respectively. These values reflect the need for heavier smoothing in smaller samples. The allocation of the 154 cases produced by the kernel method is given in Table (4(b) and is comparable with that obtained from the linear discriminant method.

Several methods are available for examining the trustworthiness or reliability of allocation probabilities [7]. Formal tests of significance are inappropriate because of the lack of an independent test set, and instead a graphical method was selected. Ideally one would examine large numbers of vibration episodes with identical signal characteristics to ensure that the distribution across the clinical groups did not deviate from that expected from the allocation probabilities. For example, if the allocation probability that such a signal was a safe click was 0.9, then this probability would be reliable if 90 out of every 100 such signals actually were safe clicks. However, such an approach is rarely practicable.

Actual	(a) Predicted			(b) Predicted		
	Normal	Click	Unstable	Normal	Click	Unstable
Normal	11	5	0	12	4	0
Click	4	129	0	7	126	0
Unstable	0	2	3	0	1	4

Table 4 Actual and predicted group membership for 154 hips using (a) linear discriminant analysis and (b) kernel discrimination.

In the current context the graphical method considers each of the 462 (154 cases X 3 groups) allocation probabilities as shots, 154 of which are hits and the remaining 308 misses. A hit is obtained only if the allocation probability is that corresponding to the actual clinical group. Allocation probabilities for the other two clinical groups are misses. If the allocation probabilities are perfectly reliable, then for any subset of shots the number of hits expected is obtained simply by adding the probabilities in the subset. Any tendency for allocation probabilities to be over-confident (i.e. too near the extremes of 0 and 1) results in small allocation percentages being hits too often. The graph is obtained by ordering the 462 allocation probabilities by size and plotting the cumulative actual hits against the cumulative expected hits. Over-confident allocation probabilities result in a plot which deviates upward from the line of equality which represents perfect reliability.

Application of this graphical reliability check resulted in the two plots shown in Figure 2. Both methods showed some tendency toward over-confidence, this being more marked for the kernel density method. The modified likelihood method has previously been noted to provide insufficient smoothing [5] and this may to some extent explain the over-confidence. The kernel density method was therefore repeated using recommendations for the smoothing parameters in the univariate normal situation based on a mean integrated square error criterion [4]. The values for the three smoothing parameters were 0.677, 0.418 and 0.903. Although there was some reduction in the over-confidence this was accompanied by a loss of discriminating power compared with that shown in Table 4(b).

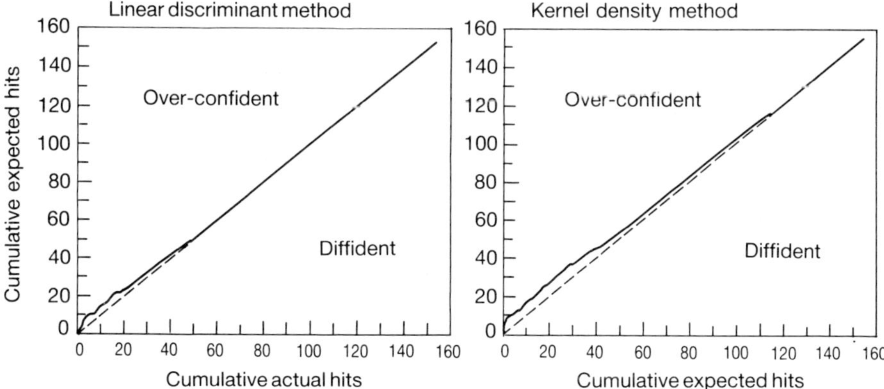

Fig. 2 Graphical reliability analysis of the allocation probabilities provided by two methods of discriminant analysis.

The linear discriminant function coefficients, after standardization through division by the pooled within group standard deviations, showed that frequency weighted most heavily on the first discriminant function. Pulse area and RMS acceleration weighted heavily but with opposite sign on both discriminant functions. In view of the high correlation known to exist between these two variables it seemed likely that the solution was unstable and that the discriminant functions might therefore perform poorly when applied to new data. RMS acceleration, the last variable to be chosen by the stepwise selection procedure, was therefore removed from the discriminant analysis. The predicted group membership did not alter from that shown in Table 4(a). A noteworthy advantage of this modification is that the results can be plotted in the space of the two chosen variables (Figure 3), and that such a plot is much more acceptable to clinicians than is a plot in the space formed by the discriminant functions. The allocation regions for the linear discriminant analysis are shown by the solid lines in Figure 3. The corresponding allocation regions for the kernel density method restricted to these same two variables are shown by the broken lines. It is clear that the two methods provide a very similar allocation rule.

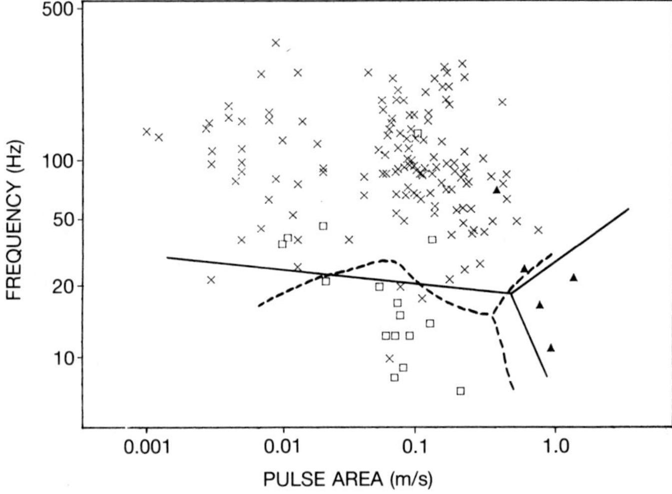

Fig. 3 Allocation regions obtained by the linear discriminant function method (———) and the kernel density estimation method (-----).

☐ = Normal X = Safe click ▲ = Unstable

5. DISCUSSION

Vibration arthrometry is a non-invasive method of detecting and recording clicks and clunks from the neonatal hip. Whilst more than 600 episodes of vibration have been reported there were smaller numbers of cases in the normal and unstable groups than is desirable. To a large extent this is an inevitable consequence of the low incidence of the condition. Nevertheless our ability to emulate the expert examiner was satisfactory with an overall correct classification rate of 93%. As had been anticipated, our discriminant analysis was unable to differentiate the safe click and CDH click groups, six of the seven signals in the latter group being allocated to the safe click group and the remaining signal to the unstable group.

Although we have used the training set to assess discriminating power, we have employed leaving-one-out methods for allocation so our results should be only slightly optimistic. Of course the clinical selection of cases was not random and our prior probabilities do not reflect the relative frequencies of the groups in the population. When these relative frequencies are available to us we will be able to incorporate them, together with estimates of the costs of misallocation, to produce a clinically relevant screening tool.

The cases for whom no signal was recorded cannot benefit from the diagnostic potential of vibration arthrometry but neither will such cases be detected by the experienced examiner.

The reproducibility of the variables may reflect the lack of control in the performance of the stress test and physical reasons for this are clear. Both magnitude and direction of the applied force during testing are variable. The mechanical support of the infant is another factor which will contribute to the inherent variability. Future work directed at standardising these factors as much as possible would be worthwhile.

The impression given of distinct clinical groups to some extent belies the continuous nature of this condition which, like most diseases, has a spectrum of severity. The equivocal nature of the groups is illustrated by the fact that the badly misallocated unstable hip shown in Figure 3, though diagnosed as unstable by the expert examiner, did not at any stage require treatment for CDH.

A further 3000 consecutive neonatal examinations have been peformed in order to validate the technique. These recordings are in the process of being analysed and the review of these children at 4 years of age is under way.

In parallel with this research an engineering project has been completed which implements the method of neonatal vibration arthrometry. The Belfast Hip Screener (Figure 4) is a computer-based screening system which dispenses with the hardware described above. The normal stress test is performed and the results stored by the computer. Signals are displayed allowing rapid time windowing, Fourier analysis and diagnostic information to be provided.

The final assessment of the clinical impact of vibration arthrometry in the early detection of CDH must await the performance of a large scale randomised trial.

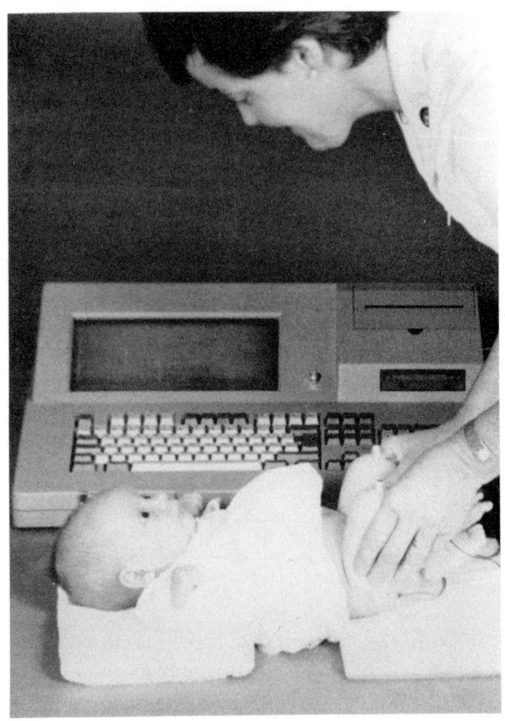

Fig. 4 A commercial package for the early detection of congenital dislocation of the hip - The Belfast Hip Screener.

6. REFERENCES

[1] Barlow, T.G., (1962) Early diagnosis and treatment of congenital dislocation of the hip, Journal of Bone and Joint Surgery 44B, 292-301.

[2] Dixon, W. J., (1983) "BMDP Statistical Software", University of California Press, Berkeley.

[3] Dunn, P. M., Evans, R. E., Thearle, M. J., Griffiths, H. E. D., and Witherow, P. J. (1985) Congenital dislocation of the hip: early and late diagnosis and management compared, Archives of Disease in Childhood, 60, 407-414.

[4] Fryer, M. J. (1976) Some errors associated with the non-parametric estimation of density functions, Journal of the Institute of Mathematics and its Applications, 18, 371-380.

[5] Fryer, M. J. (1977) A review of some non-parametric methods of density estimation, Journal of the Institute of Mathematics and its Applications, 20, 335-354.

[6] Habbema, J. D. F., Hermans, J., and Van den Broek, K. (1974) A stepwise discriminant analysis program using density estimation, in "Compstat 1974" (ed. Bruckmann, G.), Physica Verlag, Vienna.

[7] Hilden, J., Habbema, J. D. F. and Bjerregaard, B. (1978) The measurement of performance in probabilistic diagnosis. ii Trustworthiness of the exact values of the diagnostic probabilities. Methods of Information in Medicine, 17, 227-237.

[8] Kendall, M., Stuart, A., and Ord, J. K. (1983) "The Advanced Theory of Statistics (Volume 3)", Chapter 44 Classification: Discrimination and Clustering, 4th edition, Griffin, London.

[9] Plaice, M. J., Parkin, D. M. and Fitton, J. M. (1978) Effectiveness of neonatal screening for congenital dislocation of the hip. Lancet, ii, 249-250.

7. ACKNOWLEDGEMENTS

The authors wish to acknowledge the financial support of the Medical Research Council, Action Research for the Crippled Child and the Eastern Health and Social Services Board. The work could not have been completed without medical support from Mr. G. H. Cowie, MD, FRCS and staff nurses B. A. Bogues, G. E. M. Nugent, P. Walker and B. Trainor. We also thank DHSS (N.I.) for granting access to Child Health Record information.

PROBLEMS OF PROGNOSIS IN SEVERE HEAD INJURIES USING DISCRIMINANT ANALYSIS TECHNIQUES

D. Jerwood
(School of Mathematical Sciences, University of Bradford)

D.J. Price
(Department of Neurosurgery, Pinderfields Hospital, West Yorkshire)

and

F.A. Georgiakodis
(University of Piraeus, Greece)

The treatment of severe head injuries has aroused medical interest since the time of Hippocrates. At present it has been estimated that the UK annual total of "avoidable deaths" from potentially treatable complications following head injury stands at 700. Each year the Neurosurgical Department at a West Yorkshire hospital admits on average one hundred such injuries into their wards, where they are routinely assessed, investigated, monitored and optimally managed. Details such as cause of injury, pupillary and motor signs and operative findings all provide useful information for accurate prognosis.

Linear discriminant analysis techniques result generally in logistic group membership probability profiles and the risk of development of a potentially lethal haematoma can be accurately assessed within hours of admission and long before the classical symptoms of deterioration are manifest. Prompt anticipation of complications should lead ultimately to decreased mortality and morbidity. Stable discriminators which characterise good recovery or the detection of the developing haematoma are readily available. The associated rules consistently exhibit Efficiency in excess of 90%, although perhaps due medical caution is better reflected by controlling Specificity. Studies indicate that discriminant rules developed from training data provided by more severely injured patients perform equally well when applied to *apparently mild* head injuries.

Search for second-order interactive contributions leads to widespread infiltration of unstable discriminators, many of which describe interaction specifically with the referral pattern, which individually harbours no predictive potential for either diagnosis (of haematoma) or prognosis. The anticipated reduction in the zone of ambiguity, containing those patients of unclear prognosis, is far from dramatic. Evidence from a three-way discrimination, which attempts to characterise and identify the difficult group of patients who recover but with a degree of disability, strongly suggests that the group centroids are collinear and consequently all three groups may be calibrated on the same discriminant scale.

1. INTRODUCTION

Since the time of Hippocrates, much medical interest has been expressed in the problems concerned with the prognosis and treatment of head injuries. In 460 BC Hippocrates stated "No head injury is so mild that it can be ignored, nor so severe that life should be despaired of" and his observation is equally relevant today, although obviously the management of neuronal insults has changed radically. Nevertheless the attitude of many neurosurgeons in the recent past has been to offer help to those patients whose deterioration in conscious level is already manifest: consequently leading to an unacceptably high proportion of late diagnoses of complications with associated increases in morbidity and mortality rates. It has been estimated (Price, 1983) that possibly some 700 avoidable deaths occur in the UK annually from such traumatic injuries.

In recent years with every 100,000 head of population, approximately 2,500 each year will sustain a head injury, although few of them will suffer permanent brain damage as a result. Some 15 of these will be admitted to intensive care units with perhaps two or three patients sustaining multiple injuries including an "apparently mild" head injury (Miller and Jones, 1985). As Price (1985) points out, the remaining 12 or so patients either exhibit evidence of severe brain damage or have a high probability of progressive neuronal damage due to a potentially reversible secondary event. The efforts of an intensive care unit are concentrated on early prevention, recognition and rapid reversal of these secondary neuronal insults.

In 1974 Teasdale and Jennett evolved the Glasgow Coma Scale: a clinical assessment of the depth and duration of coma and grades of impaired consciousness based on independent measures of pupillary, motor and verbal responses. Subsequently Jennett and Bond (1975) assessed the outcome after severe brain damage according to the Glasgow Outcome Scale (G.O.S.) with five categories (see Table 1). Several excellent pioneering papers were published at this time generated by the Glasgow study; notably those by Jennett et al. (1976), Price and Knill-Jones (1979) and Habbema et al. (1979) and later the classic paper by Titterington et al. (1981). However each study appears to be confined to a particular category of head-injury with prognosis being attempted on a time scale measured in days rather than hours.

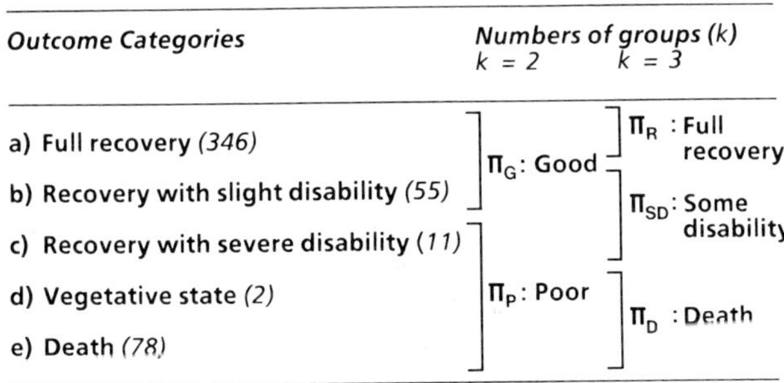

Outcome Categories	*Numbers of groups (k)* $k = 2$	$k = 3$
a) Full recovery *(346)*	Π_G: Good	Π_R : Full recovery
b) Recovery with slight disability *(55)*		Π_{SD}: Some disability
c) Recovery with severe disability *(11)*	Π_P: Poor	
d) Vegetative state *(2)*		Π_D : Death
e) Death *(78)*		

Table 1 Outcome categories for 492 severe head injuries in Pinderfield's training data and definition of sub-populations for k-group discrimination.

Frequencies given in parentheses

Between 1976 and 1980 a database consisting of observations from a series of 492 patients with severe head injury was being compiled prospectively by neurosurgeons at Pinderfields Hospital. The analysis was to search *inter alia* for criteria by which the potential for recovery could be recognised within 24 hours of the traumatic event, using a much greater variety of feature variables and whose application would be to a much wider class of head injury. The patients in the training set have been classified initially according to their outcome on the full G.O.S., although for practical purposes accurate predictions are usually considered feasible only in the two-category situation with Π_G: Good outcome and Π_P: Poor outcome.

The medical implications of this study are described by Jerwood et al. (1988a) and the present article will address the mathematical preparation of those feature variables for discrimination and a discussion of some of the aspects of the Statistical package used in the analysis. Other possible predictive targets of some medical importance include those patients harbouring a developing haematoma and the more ambitious prognosis with three categories of outcome, namely Π_R: Full recovery, Π_{SD}: Recovery with some disability and Π_D: Death or vegetative state (see Table 1). These will be discussed briefly.

2. THE PINDERFIELDS DATABASE

The full set of 21 feature variables adopted for routine monitoring is listed in Table 2. Several of these variables have appeared in previous studies, but the list has been augmented by clinical and neurosurgical signs which are available within 24 hours of injury. Complex neurological assessments were purposely excluded in order to eliminate individual subjective observer error. The variables tabulated consist of a mixture of binary (b), discrete (d) and continuous (c) observations and in the final column the results of significance tests for between-category differences are described. These initial investigations are encouraging with only five feature variables failing to exhibit any predictive potential for a patient's outcome category. Note in particular that, of the two types of fracture described in the database, the vault fracture appears irrelevant, as do the two variables associated with the referral pattern (REF and RT).

Variable	*Type*	*Brief description*	*Between-group sig.level*
SEX	b	Sex of patient	0.008
AGE	c	Age of patient	<0.001
REF	b	Local or distant referral	0.816
CI	d	Cause of injury	<0.001
FCL	d	First conscious level	<0.001
LCL	d	Later conscious level	<0.001
CLT	d	Conscious level trend	<0.001
TIA	c	Time from injury to admission	0.052
RT	c	Referral time	0.317
IPS	d	Initial pupil score	<0.001
LPS	d	Later pupil score	<0.001
PST	d	Pupil score trend	0.002
HS	d	Hemiparesis score	0.091
RHA	b	Reported headache	<0.001
SZR	b	Seizures	0.042
VF	b	Vault fracture	0.961
BF	b	Base fracture	<0.001
MLS	d	Mid-line shift	0.037
LTH	d	Laterality of haematoma	<0.001
TPH	d	Type of haematoma	<0.001
SZH	d	Size of haematoma	<0.001

Table 2 Brief description of feature variables available and results of significance tests for between-group variation.
Variable type encoded b: binary, d: discrete, c: continuous

This mixture of data types is typical of complex medical surveys with the presence of dichotomous (binary) responses, nominal (categorical) data, discrete and continuous variates and is perhaps best analysed using Fisher's linear discriminant function (Krzanowski, 1977). The majority of the variables available appear on ordinal scales, but ideally each needs to be transformed to a higher level (interval scale) before its full discriminant potential can be realised.

Binary variables are virtually by default measured on an interval scale, but as a variable assumes greater support it becomes essential to examine the response levels of the presence of an interval scale. The procedure is illustrated in Table 3 for the variable CI: Cause of injury, which has nine response levels and generates categorical data. The initial ranking could well prove numerically meaningless in any prognostic analysis.

A useful criterion for transforming ranks uses the observed mortality rates, which by good fortune exhibit a high degree of correlation with the initial ranks with only sporting accidents being conspicuously misplaced. These tranformed ranks would constitute an ordinal scale, but to register the actual observed mortality rate would be acceptable as a *prognostic* interval scale (not necesarily identical to a *diagnostic* interval scale for the prediction of the developing haematoma).

Accident Type			*Observed Mortality (%)*
Road Traffic Accident	**1**	Pedestrian	31
	2	Car	25
	3	Motor Cycle	28
	4	Cycle	17
General Accident	**5**	Industrial	18
	6	Domestic	16
	7	Sport	0
Other	**8**	Assault	12
	9	Unknown	0

Table 3 Response levels of CI : Cause of injury and observed mortality rates

Of the continuous variables examined all were presented on an ordinal scale, however LCL: Later conscious level exhibited a marked degree of limitation in the recovery profile, which was rendered linear by introducing a logarithmic transformation. Consequently LCL has ordinal response levels, but ℓnLCL is measured on an interval scale.

3. THE CLASSICAL DISCRIMINATION METHOD

Fisher's linear discrimination function can be applied without any distributional assumptions concerning the observations generated by the two patient outcome categories, Π_G and Π_P. That linear combination, which ensures maximum separation between the two category centroids, assigns a discriminant score according to Anderson's classification statistic

$$z = (\bar{\underset{\sim}{x}}_G - \bar{\underset{\sim}{x}}_P)' S_u^{-1} (\underset{\sim}{x} - \tfrac{1}{2}(\bar{\underset{\sim}{x}}_G + \bar{\underset{\sim}{x}}_P)), \tag{1}$$

where x denotes the observations associated with the patient; $\bar{\underset{\sim}{x}}_G$ and $\bar{\underset{\sim}{x}}_P$ denote centroids of good and poor outcomes respectively within the training set and S_u the unbiased estimate of the (common) variance-covariance matrix. Although Fisher's approach can be regarded as a distribution-free technique, if multivariate normality of the observations is assumed then the method is optimal and the distribution of the true discriminant function is given by $N(\pm \tfrac{1}{2}\delta^2, \delta^2)$ for patients whose outcome categories are Π_G or Π_P respectively (see Fig. 1).

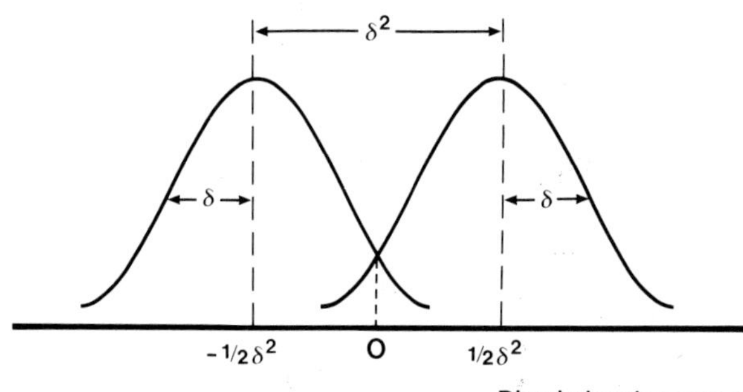

Fig. 1 Classical configuration for multivariate normal feature variables.

All the useful characteristics of these discriminant distributions may be described by the Mahalanobis (squared) distance δ^2, where

$$\delta^2 = (\underset{\sim}{\mu}_G - \underset{\sim}{\mu}_P)' \Sigma^{-1} (\underset{\sim}{\mu}_G - \underset{\sim}{\mu}_P) \tag{2}$$

and $\underset{\sim}{\mu}_G$, $\underset{\sim}{\mu}_P$ and Σ denote the analogous population centroids and common variance-covariance matrix. In particular notice that the inter-centroid distance (δ^2) is identical to the common variance of the univariate normal distributions, so that this parameter implicitly controls the extent to which overlapping occurs and consequently the Zone of Ambiguity: that is the region of discriminant scores corresponding to head injuries with uncertain prospects. Using the zero score as the critical value for allocation (corresponding to discrete uniform Bayesian priors and equal misallocation costs) yields equal error rates of magnitude $\Phi(-\frac{1}{2}\delta)$. It is easily shown that under such circumstances the conditional probability that a patient whose discriminant score is z being allocated to outcome category Π_G is logistic in structure.

In reality of course head-injured patients whatever their outcome category do not generate observations which are multivariate normal. A formal significance test proposed by Mardia (1970) is based on generalisations of skewness (using the Mahalanobis angle between each pair of corrected observations) and kurtosis (using the Mahalanobis squared distance) produces evidence against multivariate normality. Box's M-criterion may be used to test equality of the variance-covariance matrices, however it is well known that such tests are extremely sensitive to non-normality in the univariate case and this same sensitivity extends to multivariate situations. More recently Hawkins (1981) has demonstrated a novel method for the simultaneous testing of multivariate normality and equality of variance-covariance matrices.

Schematic representation of all 21 feature variables (Fig. 2) indicates the availability of each observation in real time as recorded from the patient's impact time. This time axis extends over some 24 hours and, although every feature variable is available for prognosis, for the associated problem of diagnostic discrimination for risk of a secondary event, a selection taboo should be placed on all three variables monitored during the post-operative period.

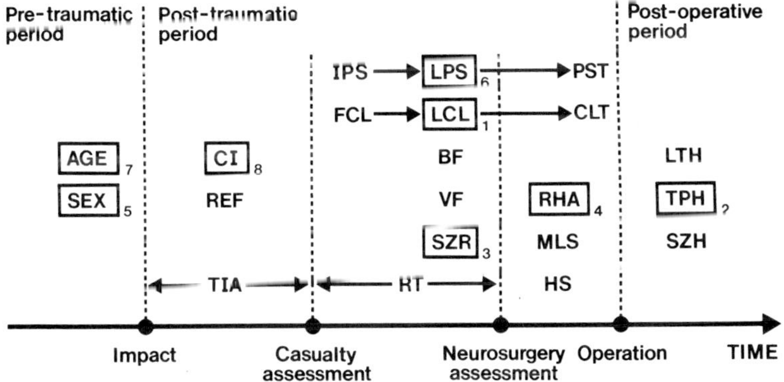

Fig. 2 Schematic representation of 21 feature variables against patient's time-event axis

Note also that the clinical signs relating to pupillary response and assessment of conscious level have been recorded both at casualty and again at neurosurgery, following the referral time period (RT). These two assessments have been differenced to produce trend values PST and CLT and such variables will inevitably lead to a degree of instability.

A stable discriminator is assigned a discriminant coefficient, whose sign agrees with the corresponding difference between category means and its interpretation is largely unequivocal. Unstable discriminators on the other hand introduce conflicting evidence in this respect and are often excluded from the variable selection procedure, since they are difficult to interpret in any rational way. Nevertheless unstable discriminators can arise in practice and are usually thought to be a consequence of the effects of multicollinearity of very unequal variance-covariance matrices (Taffler, 1982). Earlier Morrison (1969) implicated highly correlated variables as a possible source of instability.

The two clinical measurements of trend clearly introduce multicollinearity into the database, however their permitted inclusion was deliberate in order to determine whether prognostic potential was lodged with individual variable responses or with the associated trend between assessment points. Furthermore, since Box's M = 617.68 proves highly significant for this database, other sources of instability may well be anticipated.

4. SELECTION OF STABLE DISCRIMINATORS FOR GOOD OUTCOME

There are several statistical packages currently available for discriminant analyses, although none with an integrated facility for checking for unstable discriminators. Using BMDP an initial selection chose 18 of the 21 feature variables presented and these are ranked in Table 4 according to the magnitude of their standardised coefficients.

Feature Variable	Standardised Coefficients Initial Selection	Final Selection
LCL	0.45	2.28 *
AGE	- 0.30	- 0.013
RHA	- 0.29	- 0.36
TPH	- 0.27	- 0.49
IPS	0.25	-
LPS	0.23	0.24
SZR	- 0.21	- 0.37
MLS	0.18 †	-
LTH	0.14 †	-
SEX	- 0.10	- 0.27
PST	- 0.085 †	-
CLT	0.082 †	-
BF	0.070 †	-
SZH	- 0.069 †	-
CI	- 0.065	- 0.007
VF	- 0.048 †	-
HS	0.047 †	-
REF	0.033 †	-

Table 4 **Search for stable discriminators for good recovery**

† Unstable choice in initial selection
* Calibration on logarithmic scale

4.1 *Rejected Variables*

TIA, RT: Those time intervals between impact time and assessments at casualty and neurosurgery (see Fig. 2). Their rejection is not wholly surprising as no significant prognostic information was discovered here during the initial investigation (Table 2).

FCL: This initial assessment of conscious level has considerable prognostic potential, but duplicates information lodged at the more powerful later assessment of the same clinical symptoms, LCL; even though at this stage such an assessment is registered on the inferior ordinal (arithmetic) scale.

4.2 *Unstable Discriminators*

PST, CLT: These trend variables by definition introduce multicollinearity and have been already anticipated as sources of instability.

LTH, SZH: Haematoma characteristics which are highly correlated with TPH: Type of haematoma, as registered on the ordinal scale - extradural, subdural, intracerebral and mixed. It is interesting that there is more prognostic potential lodged with the *type* of haematoma than the more numerically structured *size* of haematoma.

MLS, HS: Scores relating to externally generated manifestations of the developing intracerebral haematoma. Although the links are more tenuous, these variables clearly belong to this haematoma group and are again highly correlated with TPH.

VF, REF: The binary responses are demonstrably weak (see Table 2). Their selection is perhaps surprising, however they have been relegated to relatively low positions in the discriminant rankings. With reference to the results of Table 2, it is worth emphasising that whether a patient was local or a distant referral had little influence for their prospects for long-term recovery.

4.3 Stable Discrimination

Removal of these various sources of instability and re-presenting variables for selection by BMDP will lead to a discriminant rule based entirely on stable contributions which is 91.7% efficient using the resubstitution method (91.5% efficient on Jackknife). Registering the leading discriminant (LCL) on an interval (logarithmic) scale will yield an enhanced efficiency of 93.2% and cause ℓnLCL to dominate the final selection rankings (see final column of Table 4). The corresponding stable discriminant function (or so-called canonical variable) is that advocated for calibration of the severity of a head injury.

Individual components, which contribute to this stable discriminant function, have been boxed for ease of identification in the schematic representation of Fig. 2 and each box has been indexed by the associated ranking of its standardised coefficient. Most of these discriminators have been discussed earlier, however note that both variables AGE and SEX, which are available during the pre-traumatic period, can influence final outcome with young females having the greatest potential for good recovery.

The remaining choices, namely SZR: Seizures and RHA: Reported headache are interesting, insomuch that it is the presence of both these binary responses which proves conducive to good recovery. These apparent anomalies may be explained in terms of variable surrogation, since the absence of seizures could well be due to depth of coma (rather than the injury being mild) and to report a headache requires a patient to receive and respond coherently to a verbal prompt. Hence neither variable is naturally dichotomous, nevertheless even in its present binary form each enjoys a high ranking as a stable discriminator.

5. LOGISTIC ALLOCATION PROFILES

As mentioned earlier in Section 3 a natural consequence of multivariate normality of feature variables is a logistically structured profile for allocation probabilities or equivalently linear log-odds against survival. In practice however a pre-requisite for the logistic curve

$$\Pr(\Pi_G|z) = \{1 + \exp[\alpha + \beta z]\}^{-1} \tag{3}$$

to provide a reasonable model to assess the potential for good outcome based on discriminant score z is that the generated scores be (univariate) normally distributed within each category of patient. This condition need not be satisfied globally, but is required to prevail only over the zone of ambiguity. Hence typically normal tail behaviour over this central interval is sufficient to generate allocation profiles of logistic form (3).

In Fig. 3 these allocated scores have been displayed in the usual transformed cumulative Gaussian form replacing the familiar sigmoid curves with linear plots. This graphical evidence suggests that normality is not unreasonable and formal significance tests based on both D'Agostino's Y Statistic and the modified Kolmogorov-Smirnov test reinforce this view.

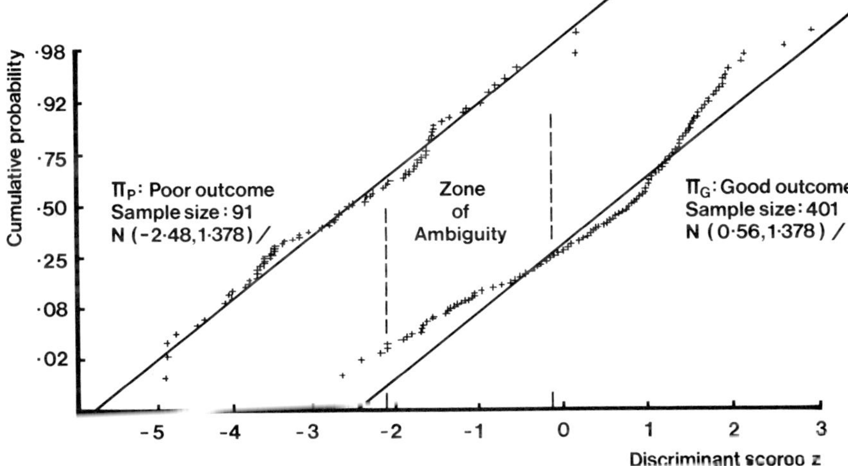

Fig. 3 Comparison of observed discrimination scores against transformed cumulative normal profiles.

This induced univariate normality is not so surprising, since linear discriminant scores are constructed as a combination of several (standardised) variates as shown by equation (1). Furthermore the parallelism of the maximum likelihood normal plots of Fig. 3 suggests that these distributions share a common variance, whose pooled estimate is 1.378. In passing note that should significantly different variances be present in these plots, then one need simply introduce an additional quadratic term into the exponential of equation (3). The horizontal displacement between these parallel plots indicates an inter-centroid distance of 3.04, which implies that in practice the degree of separation enjoyed in prognosis of severe head injuries is far in excess of that anticipated in the classical configuration described in Fig. 1. As a consequence the zone of ambiguity will be greatly reduced and the usual error rates based on $\Phi(-\frac{1}{2}\delta)$ are likely to give pessimistic estimates of misallocation.

The prognosis of patients whose discriminant scores are positive or are below -2 seem reasonably clear, but those whose scores lie within this central interval have uncertain prospects. Within the constraint imposed by the choice of the original feature variables in the database, this zone of ambiguity has been minimised by constructing that discriminant score which maximises the magnitude of the β parameter in equation (3.). The estimate of the α parameter is largely arbitrary (resulting only in a horizontal translation) and has no effect on the relative ranking of patients within the training set. In Fig. 4 $\hat{\alpha} = -3.302$ to permit positive discriminant scores to correspond to almost certain prospects of good outcome.

Several techniques are available to estimate these logistic parameters, namely least-squares regression fits to plots of log-odds against good recovery or maximum likelihood procedures for multinomial data. The resulting profile to predict the potential for good outcome Π_G is found to be

$$\Pr(\Pi_G | z, L) = \{1 + \exp[-3.302 - 2.137z]\}^{-1}, \qquad (4)$$

where L denotes use of the Linear Discriminant Model. This profile is illustrated in Fig. 4 by the unbroken graph and compares favourably with observed recovery rates. Formal significance tests (such as the conventional χ^2 goodness of fit and the generalised Likelihood Ratio Test of fit) produce no evidence to reject profile (4). It may be concluded that this profile should produce a reasonably accurate estimate of a patient's potential for good outcome within 24 hours of injury.

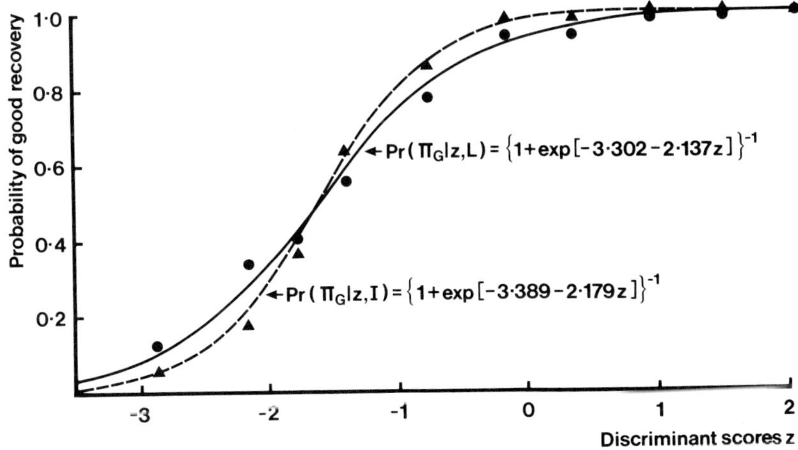

Figure 4 Logistic probability profiles for Π_G: Good recovery

——— Linear model ; ● observed rates

– – – Interaction model ; ▲ observed rates

6. THE LINEAR DISCRIMINANT PACKAGE

With the wide availability of complex statistical packages, such as those provided by BMDP and SPSS, there is an increasing need to exercise a degree of selectivity with the options available within the package. Most good statistical packages make provision for the following specifications.

(a) Calibration: An optimum scoring system producing from a multivariate input variable, $\underset{\sim}{x}$, a univariate canonical score, z. This essentially allows the patients within the training set to be ranked according to their potential for good recovery. This is the most important facility available within the procedure and the induced ranking is optimum subject to the choice of feature variables presented and their associated levels of measurement.

(b) Bayesian Prior Distribution: A probabilistic statement of *a priori* risk (p_G, p_P), which is usually difficult to assess and often defined by complete ignorance, when each outcome category is assumed initially to be equally likely.

(c) Misallocation Costs: An economic statement of the consequences of erroneous predictions (C_G, C_P). Once again these are difficult to assess accurately and often taken (with little justification) to be equal.

(d) Efficiency: A measurement of allocation success based on the percentage of correctly predicted head injuries over both categories of patients. The optimum allocation rule requires that Π_G: Good outcome be predicted, whenever the assigned discriminant score, z, satisfies

$$z \gtrless \ell n \left(\frac{p_G}{p_P} \cdot \frac{C_P}{C_G} \right). \tag{5}$$

This critical value reduces to zero, when costs are assumed equal and the Bayesian prior taken to be discrete uniform (see Fig. 1), and error rates become $\Phi(-\frac{1}{2}\delta)$.

These last three specifications of the discrimination procedure presuppose that allocation is inevitable, which is manifestly untrue. In *diagnostic* situations it is consistent to propose a course of treatment and so allocation will be a natural consequence; however in *prognostic* situations it is unlikely that management of the patient will be affected by this analysis. Hence it is more appropriate in prognosis to construct as accurate a probabilistic description of the outcome categories as possible. A comparison of the logistic probability profile with the observed recovery rates (see Fig. 4) illustrates the magnitude of the random sampling error which is inherent in any stochastic formulation. With large data sets and reasonably accurate calibration such errors should be small. However even if such sampling errors were entirely eliminated and the resulting probability profiles were to describe perfectly the potential for recovery, then the allocation procedure is unlikely to be fully efficient. Efficiency measures may therefore be influenced more by the usual risks of prediction than by the inappropriateness of the theoretical model. Fully efficient allocation can only result from total separation of the outcome categories and is seldom achieved in practice.

The search for maximum efficiency within allocation is useful only when realistic values have been assigned to both Bayesian priors and misallocation costs. More acceptable and certainly easier to implement are the group-specific measures of success, namely Sensitivity and Specificity, which allow due medical caution to be exercised. An allocation rule with a fixed level of Specificity is readily constructed directly from the profile in Fig. 4 by selection of a critical score. Within this present study profiles of total cost of misallocation exhibit little variation over the zone of ambiguity, even when there are quite large differentials between individual costs (C_G and C_p). Hence an overly cautious level of Specificity can often be justified purely on economic grounds.

7. DISCRIMINANT MODELS WITH INTERACTION TERMS

Accepting that equation (4) is optimum, no increase in accuracy of the modelling of the statistical environment can be anticipated without the introduction of extra variables, whose prognostic potential is not duplicated by those initial feature variables listed in Table 2. An alternative procedure however may be to introduce into the linear model the extra complexity of interaction terms between selected pairs of observations and defined as a product of the individual observations. When the selected observations are both binary this construction is analogous to the familiar interaction terms in ANOVA. Unlike a correlation coefficient, which essentially comments on *expected frequency* of a particular combination of variables, an interaction will describe the *consequence* to the model when those specified variables are simultaneously present.

There is little practical advice given in the literature as to a suitable introduction procedure and in the present study there are in excess of 200 possible interactions, many of which appear to have some prognostic power. Presenting some of the more powerful combinations together with the original feature variables leads to a confusing selection of discriminators. Only four of the original 21 main variables were selected, of which only SZR: Seizures was common to the two listings; the others being PST: Pupil score trend, IPS: Initial pupil score and perhaps most surprisingly REF: Local or distant referral. This last observation is known individually to harbour no prognostic potential (see Table 2) nor is it implicated in the diagnosis of haematoma complications. The remaining discriminators implicated in this model are entirely of second-order interactions and associated mainly with the referral variable, REF.

The discriminant scores may be recalculated using this Interaction model and the probability profile for the potential for good recovery (Π_G) becomes

$$\Pr(\Pi_G | z, I) = \{1 + \exp[-3.389 - 2.179z]\}^{-1} \qquad (6)$$

which is also given in Fig. 4 by the broken plot. The slight increase in the magnitude of the estimate of β leads to a moderate reduction in the zone of ambiguity and consequently an improved measure of Efficiency. However the improvement is far from dramatic in this respect. More encouraging perhaps is that the observed recovery rates are in much closer agreement with the theoretical profile and sampling errors have been virtually eliminated. Nevertheless predictions are still to be made within this stochastic environment and allocation procedures will still be far from being fully efficient. This moderate improvement however is welcome, since Murray (1977) explains that paradoxically efficiency of allocation may not necessarily be enhanced by increasing the number of variables available.

The main disadvantages inherent in this model are that several prognostically weak variables have been apparently promoted and that many of the interactions introduced into the selection procedure are highly correlated. The degree of induced stability exceeds that experienced in the initial run described in Table 4, and now there is the more serious complication that instability infiltrates even the higher-order discriminators.

8. RANGE OF APPLICATION OF THE PROGNOSTIC MODEL

The linear discriminant model described earlier, although developed specifically for prognosis of severe head injuries, has recently been applied with some success to apparently mild head injuries. It therefore has potential as a primary filter for such injuries presented at casualty departments in order to identify those patients requiring further observation. Moreover it may be reasonably argued that those stable discriminators listed in Table 4 can be applied globally for assessment of the potential for good recovery from a head injury whatever the severity (within the present predictive framework of monitoring the initial set of 21 feature variables). Dilution of a training set with mild injuries should not necessarily undermine the power to discriminate over the critical zone of ambiguity.

Similarly for the three-outcome category problem with Π_{SD} denoting those patients who would recover with some degree of disability (see Table 1; k = 3). The re-definition of patient outcome categories could conceivably implicate a second canonical variate; however the principal discriminant function is found to explain 97% of all the information associated with the data (Jerwood et al., 1988b). Consequently it may be concluded that spatially the centroids are arranged in a collinear configuration (see Lachenbruch, 1973) and we may identify these three outcome categories as manifestations of the severity of the same medical condition. Even in this more complicated diagnostic situation, patients will still be calibrated on a single discriminant scale, which is found not to differ significantly from the stable two-category prognostic scale described in Table 4. The resulting allocation probability profiles have been re-estimated based on the two-category scale and are illustrated in Fig. 5 together with the observed allocation rates. Generally there is close agreement between observed and theoretical rates - except over the lower end of the zone of ambiguity, where discrepancies appeared for patient groups Π_{SD}: Some disability and Π_D: Death (or vegetative state). These discrepancies may well be due to low frequencies of patients in such categories.

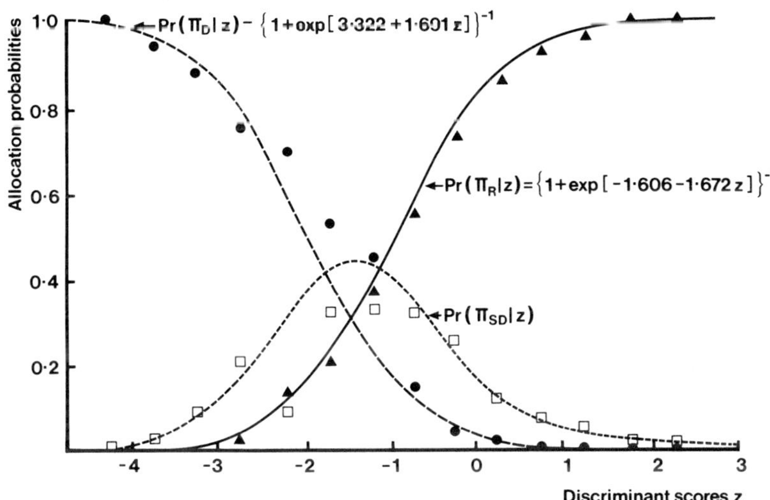

Figure 5 Final outcome probability profiles and observed rates

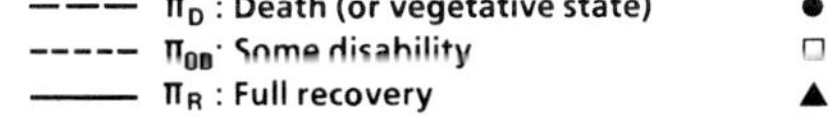

Note that only within a very narrow interval of scores will Π_{SD} (when available) prove to be the most likely prognosis. This same interval coincides with the range of scores where observed frequencies of disabilities fell noticeably below theoretical predictions. Much lower levels of efficiency are also to be anticipated in this more ambitious prognostic situation, considering the higher risks which are naturally associated with three-outcome prediction.

9. CONCLUSIONS

Complex medical data will often contain every level of variable, for which there is general agreement that a linear discriminant function should prove most suitable. In preparation for the analysis each feature variable should be presented at least on an ordinal scale and principal discriminators may be particularly sensitive and will realise their full prognostic potential only if calibrated on an interval scale.

Linear discriminant scores will often be normally distributed across each outcome category of patient, which will lead naturally to logistic allocation probability profiles. Should variances also be significantly different for each outcome category, then the log-odds of good recovery, expressed in terms of the discriminant score, z, are no longer linear but require an additional quadratic contribution. It is unnecessary however that normality should be induced globally, since logistically structured profiles can be produced by restricted induction of normality only over the central zone of ambiguity.

By far the most important facility within the discriminant package is calibration, by which the training data are optimally ranked by their multivariate symptoms complexes suitably transformed to a univariate scale. Sources of instability within the databank should be identified and removed and the introduction of interaction terms approached by a forward-selection procedure or guided by some *a priori* considerations.

Once important stable discriminators have been selected for severe head injuries, then it would seem reasonable to expect successful discrimination with apparently mild head injuries on the same discriminant scale. This same discriminant scale may even prove useful for prediction in the three-outcome category situation, where the central category of patient is seldom found to be the most likely prognosis.

REFERENCES

Habbema, J.D.F., Braakman, R. and Avezaat, C.J.J., (1979) Prognosis of the individual patient with severe head injury. Acta Neurochirurgica Supplement 28, 158-60.

Hawkins, D.M., (1981) A new test for multivariate normality and homoscedasticity. Technometrics 23, 105-10.

Jennett, B. and Bond, M., (1975) Assessment of outcome after severe brain damage. Lancet i, 480-4.

Jennett, B., Teasdale, G. and Braakman, R. et al., (1976) Predicting the outcome in individual patients after severe head injury. Lancet i, 1031-4.

Jerwood, D., Price, D.J. and Georgiakodis, F.A., (1988a) Predicting the potential for recovery within 24 hours of a head injury. University of Bradford Research Report SOR 88-24.

Jerwood, D., Price, D.J. and Georgiakodis, F.A., (1988b) Prognosis in the case of three outcome categories of patient with application to head injuries. University of Bradford Research Report SOR 88-25.

Krzanowski, W.J., (1977) The performance of Fisher's linear discriminant function under non-optimal conditions. Technometrics, 19, 191-200.

Mardia, K.V., (1970) Measures of multivariate skewness and kurtosis with applications. Biometrika, 57, 519-30.

Miller, J.D. and Jones, P.A., (1985) The work of a regional head injury service. Lancet i, 1141-4.

Morrison, M.G., (1969) On the interpretation of discriminant analysis. Journal of Marketing Research, 6, 156-63.

Murray, G.D., (1977) A cautionary note on selection of variables in discriminant analysis. Applied Statistics, 26, 246-50.

Price, D.J., (1983) A comparative study of the haematoma predictive capabilities of clinical and radiological features. In Fenton Lewis, A. (ed.) The Management of Acute Head Injury, London DHSS (Harrogate Seminars 8), 77-82.

Price, D.J., (1985) Principles of managing intracranial injuries. Care of the Critically Ill, 1, 3-5.

Price, D.J. and Knill-Jones, R.P., (1979) The prediction of outcome of patients admitted following head injury in coma with bilateral fixed pupils. Acta Neurochirurgia Supplement 28, 179-82.

Taffler, R.J., (1982) Forecasting company failure in the UK using discriminant analysis and financial ratio data. J.R. Statist. Soc., A, 40, 342-58.

Teasdale, G. and Jennet, B., (1974) Assessment of coma and impaired consciousness. Lancet ii, 81-4.

Titterington, D.M., Murray, G.D. and Murray, L.S. et al., (1981) Comparison of discrimination techniques applied to a complex data set of head injured patients. J.R. Statist. Soc. A, 144, 145-75.

RISK FACTOR ANALYSIS IN EARLY DETECTION OF BLOOD CLOTS IN ORTHOPAEDIC PATIENTS

W.G. Kernohan, P.E. Ward, F.B. Bradley, J.G. Brown, C.C. Patterson and R.A.B. Mollan

(Department of Orthopaedic Surgery, Musgrave Park Hospital, Queen's University of Belfast)

1. INTRODUCTION

Deep vein thrombosis, DVT, the formation of a blood clot in the venous system is a major problem in medicine. Of these clots, most originate in the lower limbs. There they cause chronic problems of aching legs, skin discolouration, ankle swelling and varicose ulcers. These symptoms are collectively called the post-phlebitic syndrome and occur when the obstructed vein is recanalised. Recanalisation can take from nine months to six years and the resulting veins have no valves which makes the calf muscle pump inefficient thus causing the problems associated with post phlebitic syndrome. A fragment of the thrombus can also break off and travel to the lungs there causing respiratory distress and even death. This fragment is called a pulmonary embolism and is a very serious complication of a blood clot.

Venous thrombi are very difficult to detect. Often the first sign is when the patient experiences acute respiratory distress because of a pulmonary embolism. Recent statistics show that there are 50,000 hospitalications per year in the United Kingdom due to deep vein thrombosis and 6,000 deaths per year in the United Kingdom are attributed to pulmonary embolism. When this figure is compared to the 5,800 deaths per year in the United Kingdom due to road traffic accidents the extent of the problem can be more fully appreciated. (1).

Deep vein thrombosis is a very real problem in orthopaedic surgery. It is thought that this is due to the operation sites often being on or near the lower limb and the resultant immobility in the immediate post-operative period. Workers in this field cite the DVT rate after total hip replacement in the range of 26% - 50% with pulmonary embolism rates of 1.2% - 3.5% (2,3,4).

Venography is the 'gold standard' in detecting venous thrombosis. It involves injecting a dye into the venous system of the leg via a vein in the foot. The leg is then X-rayed and any obstruction within the veins can be identified. However there are problems with venography. The test is invasive and only provides a static examination in that it gives a "snapshot" of the venous system. It is not an examination that can easily be repeated every few days and furthermore it is also a specialist technique requiring the skills of an experienced radiologist. Moreover there is also the problem that an allergic reaction can occur as a result of the dye and it is possible that the procedure may cause embolisation of an existing thrombus.

Prophylactic regimes for the prevention of DVT include the use of low dose heparin, ancrod (an extract of snake venom), dextran and aspirin. Although these have been shown to be of some use in general surgery, they are of little benefit in orthopaedic surgery. The use of anticoagulants in orthopaedic surgery leads to an increased bleeding tendency, the formation of of wound haemotomas, subsequent infection and implant failure. Physical methods for the prevention of DVT include early mobilisation, leg elevation, the wearing of graded compression stockings and recently the use of electrical calf muscle stimulation per-operatively. (5).

Since the above measures are not entirely successful in orthopaedic surgery, some method which will allow clinicians to identify those patients most likely to develop a DVT would be a considerable benefit. It was therefore decided to carry out a detailed study of orthopaedic patients to find an identification method.

2. MATERIALS AND METHODS

Eight hundred patients admitted to the Withers Orthopaedic Centre of the Musgrave Park Hospital for elective total hip replacement during the period January 1985 to December 1987 were included in the study. These patients were seen pre-operatively and on days 3, 6 and 10 post-operatively.

Pre-operative clinical factors thought to predispose a person to a blood clot were recorded along with some theatre and post-operative details. The pre-operative details included patient age, height/weight ratio, diastolic blood pressure, the presence of varicose veins, heart disease, and a previous history of DVT or PE or a family history of the same. Other data recorded included the type of anaesthesia used, the side of operation, oedema present post-operatively and the varying levels of post-operative mobility. Each patient was given a mobility score. A factor of zero indicated that the patient was bedbound, one that they could walk short distances with a walking aid, the patient was walking well with crutches for a score of two and three meant that the patient was mobile and walking well with a crutch or stick if not independently.

These details were gathered for each patient using a database package. For statistical analysis the data was transferred to a mainframe computer. A points system was developed to identify those patients likely to develop a DVT. This points system is described in Table 1 and was determined by combining published results of a literature search with the subjective view of clinicians. The distribution of variables were examined in two groups of patients; those who developed a DVT and those who did not. (6,7,8).

Figure 1 illustrates the method of impedance plethysmography involving the recording of changes in blood volume. It uses changes in the electrical impedance of the limb to assess changes in blood volume associated with the inflation and deflation of a thigh cuff. The thigh cuff is inflated to a pressure of 50mm Hg. This allows blood to flow into the leg but obstructs the venous outflow. Four electrodes are attached to the calf, two on each band. A potential difference is applied across the outer two and the changes in impedance are measured by the inner two. This is to reduce the edge effect at the electrodes. The resultant tracings are demonstrated in Figure 2. When the cuff is inflated the blood volume of the calf increases until the pressure in the calf is equal to the pressure in the cuff. This total blood volume is referred to as the venous capacitance (VC). The cuff is then released allowing the blood to flow back to the heart via the venous system. The flow of blood from the leg during the first three seconds is referred to as the venous outflow (VO). These two results can then be plotted on a graph which has a published discriminant line (the line of Hull) indicating whether the patient's blood flow is normal or whether there is an obstruction present. (9).

TABLE 1

POINTS SYSTEM FOR ASSESSING THE SUSCEPTIBILITY OF TOTAL HIP REPLACEMENT PATIENTS TO DEEP VENOUS THROMBOSIS

Clinical Variable	Points
Age: 60	0
61-70	1
71	2
Weight/obesity: 10% above mean for sex and age	1
25% above mean for sex and age	2
Rheumatoid arthritis	1
Osteoarthritis	2
Presence of varicose veins	1
Cigarette smoking	1
Use of non steroidal anti-inflammatory drugs	1
Past history of DVT/PE	3
Under transfusion of blood	1
Infected wound site	1
Late post-operative mobility	1

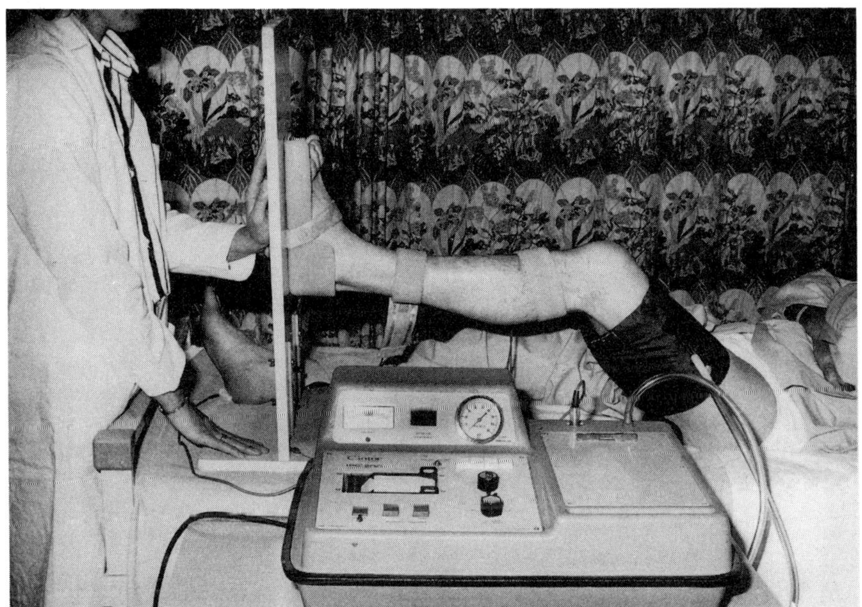

Fig. 1 Showing a patient set up for testing using the method of impedance plethysmography. A cuff is placed around the thigh allowing arterial filling, but preventing venous return. Two pairs of electrodes are attached, one at either end of the calf muscle, which monitor the impedance as the cuff is deflated. This is used to assess the venous system.

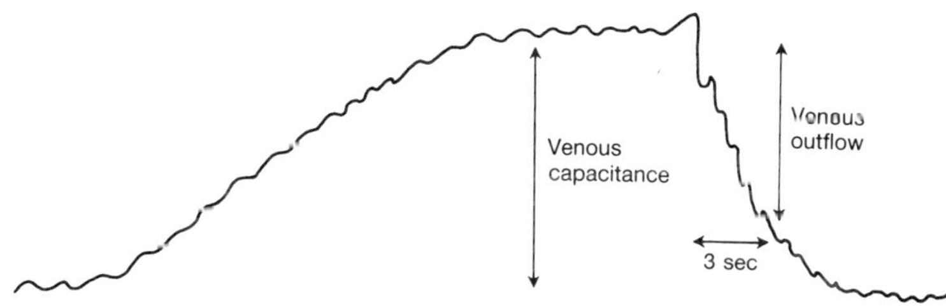

Fig. 2 Impedance plethysmograph trace from a normal subject showing venous filling after the cuff is inflated and rapid venous emptying after the cuff is deflated.

Impedance plethysmography was carried out on all 800 patients pre-operatively and on days 3, 6 and 10 post-operatively. Both legs were examined on each occasion.

3. RESULTS

When the distribution of the 'points for DVT' was examined in the two groups it was found that the points for the non DVT group were almost normally distributed about a mean of six points while the DVT group results had an excess of patients with a higher score. These distributions are illustrated in Figures 3 and 4.

A comparison of the variables in the two groups of patients is shown in Table 2. Patients who developed DVTs were almost 5 years older on average, but none of the other variables recorded pre-operatively attained statistical significance. The score for the degree of mobility for each patient on each visit gave highly significant differences between the two groups with over 60% of the DVT cases having a score of 0 or 1.

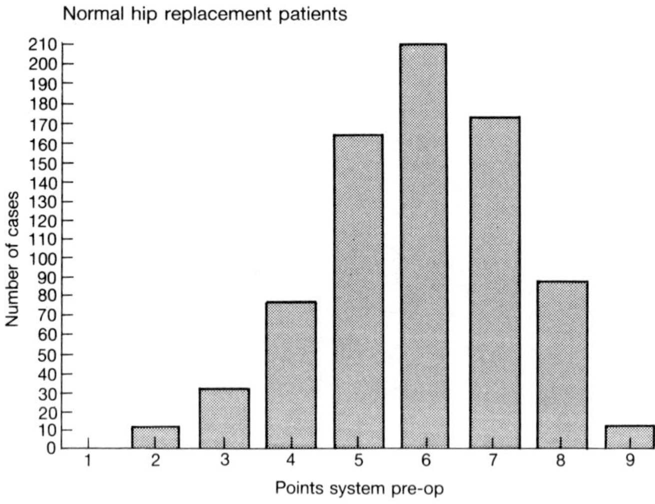

Fig. 3 The points-for-DVT in the large control group

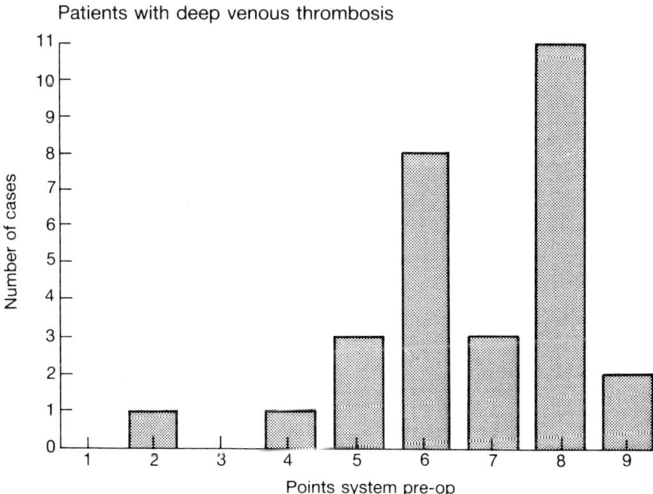

Fig. 4 The points-for-DVT in the DVT group

The presence of oedema (or swelling) on the affected side was also significant with a higher percentage of patients with oedema in the affected group.

It was expected that a combination of these clinical factors would provide better predictive value, than any single factor on its own. The clinical data was transported to GLIM with the aim of developing a new scoring method based on a multiple logistic analysis. Within GLIM it was possible to investigate the independent contribution of each variable to the discrimination. The result was a linear function of the variables which could be used to predict the probability of getting a DVT. Figure 5 illustrates the predicted probability for the control (no DVT) group. A very small number have a predicted probability of greater than 10% of developing a DVT. Figure 6 shows that there is a higher percentage of cases in the symptomatic group with a higher probability of forming a DVT. However, it is clear that 8 cases of the 29 in the DVT group have a negligible probability. In an attempt to improve the predictive value of the model the results of plethysmography have been included.

TABLE 2

COMPARISON OF THE CLINICAL FACTORS RECORDED FOR BOTH GROUPS

Variable		DVT group	Control group
Age (year)		70.4±9.1	65.9 ± 9.8
Overweight	0	17 (59%)	385 (50%)
	1	3 (10%)	217 (28%)
	2	5 (17%)	112 (15%)
	3	4 (14%)	57 (7%)
Varicose veins		12 (41%)	232 (30%)
Heart disease		13 (45%)	273 (35%)
Previous DVT/PE		3 (10%)	50 (6%)
Family history		0 (0%)	25 (3%)
Diastolic BP mmHg		85.0± 13.2	82.1 ± 11.6
Spinal anaesthesia		5 (17%)	175 (23%)
Mobility (day 2)	0	3 (10%)	66 (9%)
	1	15 (52%)	128 (17%)
	2	10 (34%)	521 (68%)
	3	1 (3%)	56 (7%)
Oedema		7 (24%)	71 (9%)
Points system	Pre-op	7	6
	Day 3	8	7
	Day 6	9	7

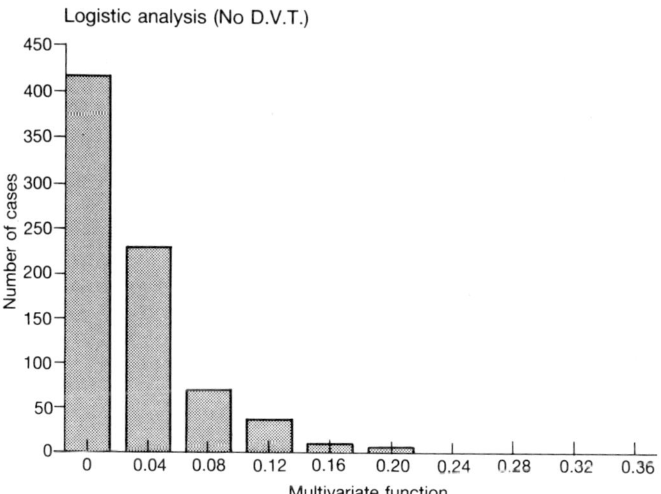

Fig. 5 The result of analysis of the control group showing the number of cases in each category of the multivariate function produced by GLIM.

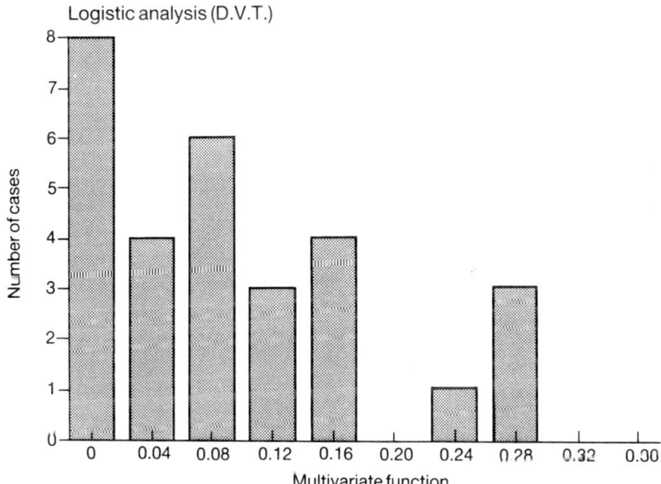

Fig. 6 In the symptomatic group the majority of cases have a non-zero probability but the minority (8) are predicted as false negatives.

Figures 7 and 8 are scattergrams of VC and VO measurements for our two groups of patients with the line of Hull superimposed. The false positive rate was 7.8% and the false negative rate 38%. These results led us to investigate the performance of VC and VO in association with the clinical factors.

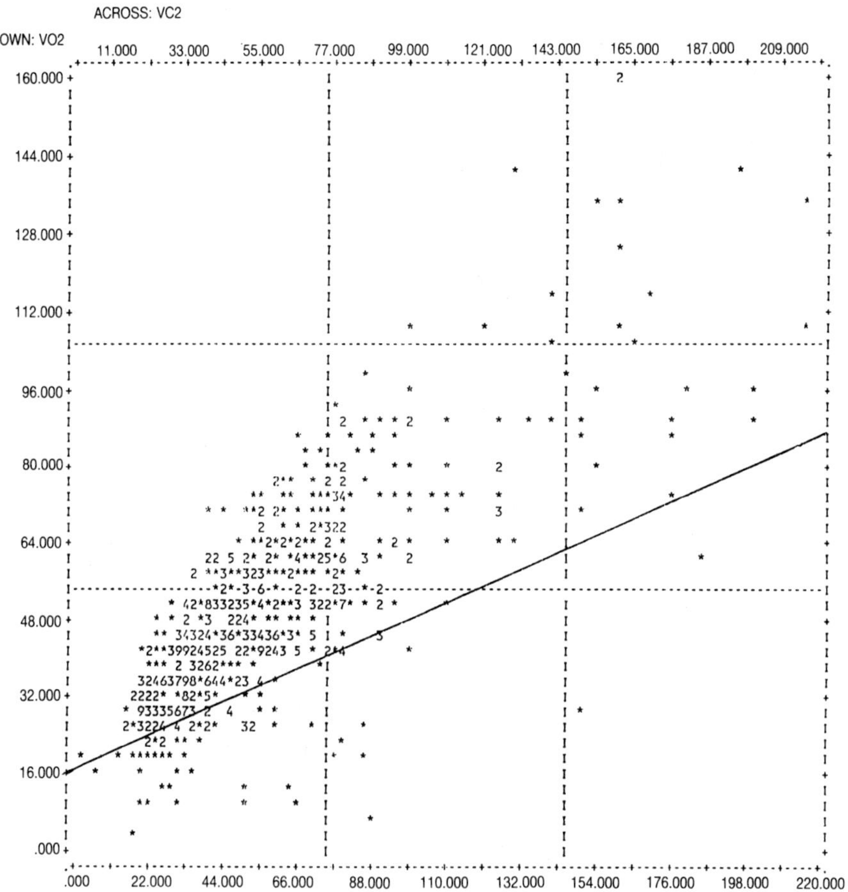

Fig. 7 When venous capacitance and outflow are used for discrimination (Hull, 9) just 7.8% of the control group are predicted to have a clot.

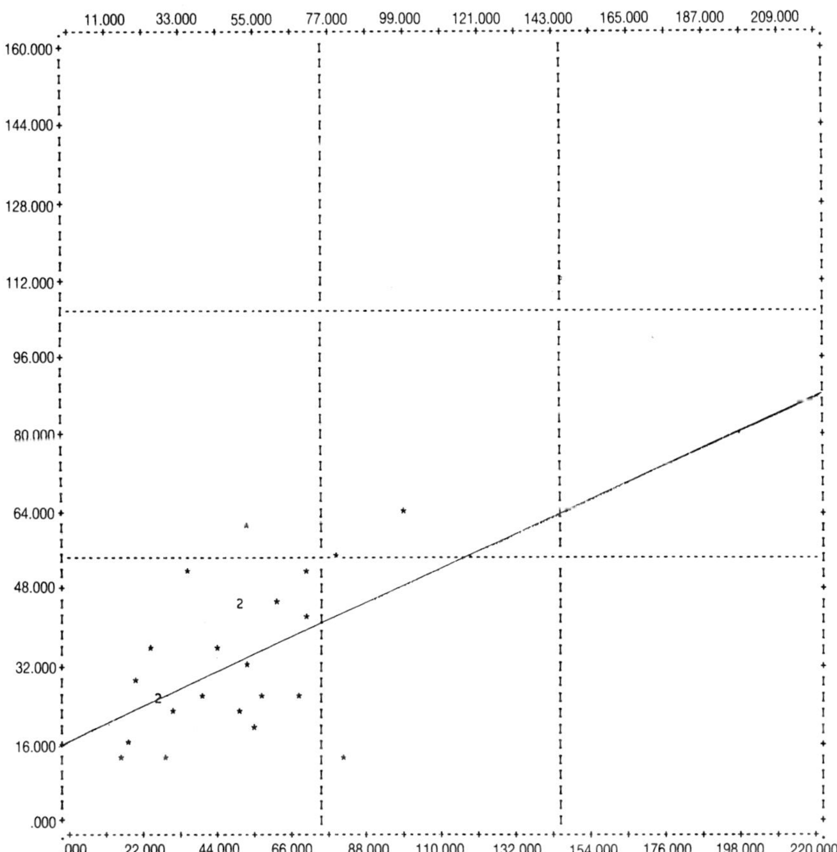

Fig. 8 The use of VC and VO in the symptomatic group give a prediction of 38% normal (false negative rate = 38%)

Tests of significance suggested that the measurements of VC and VO were helpful in indicating the patients who were developing a DVT. This is not quite the same as a predictive combination of clinical factors. The thrombus has to be forming to obtain a positive result. Table 3 shows the mean values of VC and VO for the pre-operative, days 3 and 6 visits. Often by the fourth visit the patient has been discharged and no results were available. The largest differences in means occur on the second visit, just after the operation. Both VC and VO on the operative side show significant differences on this visit. On day three VC becomes a poor indicator but VO is still indicating a difference between normal and abnormal in the operative leg. At no stage were measurements on the non-operative leg found to be a useful.

TABLE 3

AVERAGE VENOUS CAPACITANCE AND OUTFLOW MEASUREMENTS MADE PREOPERATIVELY AND TWICE POSTOPERATIVELY IN 29 PATIENTS WITH A DVT and 771 CONTROLS (ARBITRARY UNITS)

Variable	Visit	DVT Group	Controls
Right Venous Capacitance	1	56	62
	2	51	56
	3	30	59
Left Venous Capacitance	1	57	62
	2	47	54
	3	37	57
Right Venous Outflow	1	41	52
	2	42	48
	3	25	52
Left Venous Outflow	1	47	52
	2	36	47
	3	27	51

It was expected and is normal for the VC to fall after any major surgery to the lower limb, then over a period of time to recover. For the affected group the value of VC falls even lower than that seen in the control group and it is the visit first time post-operatively that was found to be the most significant. In the controls the average outflow rate drops after the operation by 6 units. By contrast the affected group shows a marked drop in outflow rate of 24 units and this would indicate that a DVT was forming. This difference is continued through until the next visit when the outflow rate is still significantly lower in the abnormal group.

In the clinical situation it is usual to compare the VC and VO of the operative leg with those for the non-operative leg. The ratio of results comparing the two legs was examined. A significant difference for VO on day 2 was shown. In the same way it is usual to compare measurements taken before the operation with those obtained in the post-operative phase. The p value for VO indicates that there is a significant difference when the first post-operative readings are compared with the pre-operative readings.

It was decided to rerun the logistic analysis, including the clinical factors together with VC and VO. The multiple logistic analysis provided a score calculated from a linear combination of VO, mobility, age and VC. When these variables were included in the model no other variables contributed significantly to the fit of the model. The final logistic scoring system is shown below:

LOGISTIC SCORING SYSTEM

$$\text{Score} = -5.3 - 0.07 \times (\text{VO}) + \begin{cases} 0 & \text{Mob} = 0 \\ +1.079 & \text{Mob} = 1 \\ -0.221 & \text{Mob} = 2,3,4 \end{cases} + 0.053 \times (\text{Age}) + 0.019 \times (\text{VC})$$

Notice that the higher the value of VO the lower the score, whilst the higher the age the higher the score. It is not clear why an intermediate value for mobility should result in a higher score. It may be that patients with a mobility score of zero are bedbound and the medical and nursing staff immediately recognise the increased risk of a clot forming and take preventive measures. A negative coefficient for VC was expected. Although this was found to be so in univariate analysis, multivariate analysis produced a positive coefficient, because of the high correlation with VO. For a given value of VO, a higher VC is associated with an increased risk.

To convert the score into a probability the equation below may be used.

$$\text{Probability} = \frac{\exp\ (\text{score})}{1 - \exp\ (\text{score})}$$

Figures 9 and 10 illustrate the results for the large control group and the smaller DVT group . As before the majority of controls have a negligible predicted probability of DVT. If the first group of the bargraph is taken as normal then, in the clinical situation, the other cases would need further examination

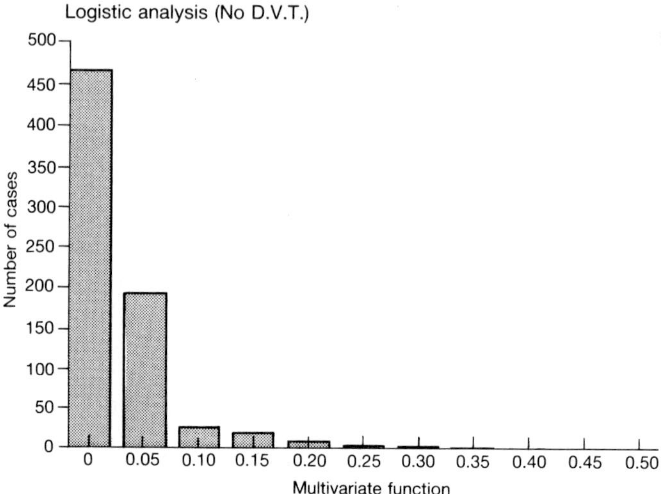

Fig. 9 Bargraph showing predicted probability of DVT in the clinically negative group (normals).

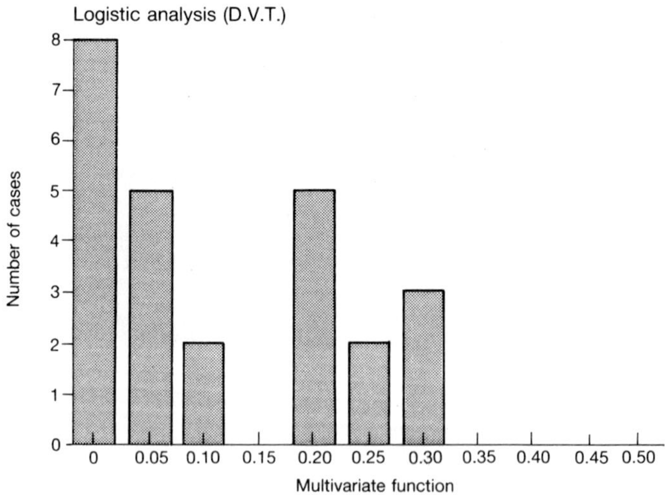

Fig. 10 Showing predicted probability of DVT in the clinically positive group.

by venography. In implementing this method as a screening procedure an arbitrary specificity of 85% will produce a sensitivity of only 48%. This would mean that 85% are being successfully cleared by the system, and 48% are being detected. If the normals were to include the first two groups of the bargraph, then there would be a specificity of 60% with a sensitivity of 68%. This might be preferable because potentially more lives are saved at the expense of a 40% venogram rate.

6. CONCLUSION

In parallel with this analysis, to implement this method suitable hardware has been developed to record VC and VO and input mobility and age. A new screener is being developed with these points in mind. It will consist of an IBM compatible computer with suitable interfaces to allow plethysmography results to be recorded, displayed and analysed. Equipment to inflate the cuff and a printer to produce a hard copy will be included. Clinical variables of value will also be inputed to the discriminant package.

In summary we have examined a group of 800 orthopaedic patients and noted clinical and impedance plethysmographic findings. Important clinical factors were mobility and age. Most significant plethysmographic readings were made on the first visit post-operatively, particularly the VO reading. Taken together these clinical factors and readings can help us to detect the at-risk patient allowing clinical preventative measures to be taken.

REFERENCES

1. Health Statistics, World Health Organisation, (1988).

2. Kakkar, V.V., Howe, C.T., Flanc, C and Clarke, M.B., (1969) Natural history of postoperative deep-vein thrombosis. Lancet; ii:230-2.

3. Crawford, W.J., Hillman, F. and Charnley, J., (1968) A clinical trial of prophylactic anticoagulant therapy in elective hip surgery. Centre for hip surgery, Wrightington Hospital: Internal publication 14.

4. Harrold, A.J., (1982) Outlook for hip replacement. Br. Med. J.; 284:139-40.

5. Kernohan, W.G., Brown, J.G., Ward, P.E. and Mollan, R.A.B., (1989) Muscle stimulation for the prevention of venous stasis during surgery. In J.P. Paul, et al (eds.), Progress in Bioengineering, Adam Hilger, Bristol. 253-5.

6. Clayton, J.K., Anderson, J.A. and McNicol, G.P., (1976) Preoperative prediction of postoperative deep vein thrombosis. Br. Med. J. 2: 910-2.

7. Crandon, A.J., Peel, K.R., Anderson, J.A., Thompson, V. and McNicol, G.P., (1980) Post-operative deep vein thrombosis: identifying high-risk patients. Br. Med. J. 281:343-5.

8. Farmer, D.A. and Smithwick, R.H., (1950) Thromboembolic Disease. Angiology; 1:191-301.

9. Hull, R., van Aken, W.G., Hirsh, J., et al., (1976) Impedance plethysmography using the occlusive cuff technique in the diagnosis of venous thrombosis. Circulation 56:696-700.

CORRESPONDENCE ANALYSIS AND INDEPENDENT BAYES FOR CLINICAL DIAGNOSIS

N.J. Crichton and J.P. Hinde
(Mathematical Statistics and Operational Research Department, University of Exeter)

ABSTRACT

The development of statistical aids for clinical diagnosis has been an area of much research in recent years. Typically a patient's symptoms are observed and by some process the probabilities of various diseases, given the patient's symptoms, are calculated. A widely used method is independent Bayes in which symptoms are assumed to be independent conditional on the disease category. Whilst in practice this assumption is unlikely to hold, the method seems to work well.

Examining the dependence between symptoms may make it possible to improve this procedure. Correspondence analysis provides one method of exploring structure in such data. Use of correspondence analysis enables us to identify clusters of symptoms showing high dependence. Selection of symptoms from different clusters provides a set more closely in line with the assumption of independent Bayes.

This paper shows the advantages of exploratory techniques as simple and quick ways of revealing the structure in symptom data and relating this to known diagnostic classifications. The methods are illustrated on data for patients attending the Accident and Emergency department complaining of chest pain.

1. INTRODUCTION

The use of probability approaches to medical diagnosis and decision making has been researched for many years. Numerous different methods of discrimination have been tried in an attempt to predict, using symptom information, the diagnosis or prognosis for the patient. Titterington et al [14] compare the merits of several discrimination techniques by applying the different methods to a set of head injured patients. Their analysis shows that none of the methods is clearly superior to the others.

One of the methods considered by Titterington et al [14] is the independent Bayes approach. This approach has been used extensively in attempts to develop clinical decision aids [3,4,12]. The results have been remarkably good despite the unrealistic assumption of symptom independence. The method has been used to develop a computerised aid for the diagnosis of acute abdominal pain [3] and a recent multicentre trial of this system has shown it to perform better than the unaided clinician [1].

The purpose of this paper is to discuss how correspondence analysis can be used to help overcome some of the problems encountered in using the independent Bayes approach. The value of using correspondence analysis in conjunction with independent Bayes will be illustrated by considering the diagnosis of patients arriving at the Accident and Emergency department (A & E) complaining of anterior chest pain. The aim of the decision aid is to identify those patients requiring admission to the coronary care unit (CCU).

The data considered in this paper is a small subset of the information collected as part of a chest pain study carried out at Westminster Hospital London. The data has been divided into two sets, 295 cases form a training set and 133 cases form a test set. For each patient 18 indicants are recorded. 16 of the indicants are nominal, most being binary. The other two indicants are ordinal (continuous variables that have been grouped). For each patient we know whether they were 'high risk cardiac' (HRC) requiring admission to CCU, or whether they were 'not high risk cardiac' (NHRC), which enables us to assess the performance of any decision rule.

2. THE INDEPENDENT BAYES APPROACH

This approach addresses the problem of differential diagnosis, assuming that the patient belongs to one of a limited number of exclusive and exhaustive categories $D_1,\ldots,D_m$. In order to make a diagnosis the doctor observes a number of symptoms exhibited by the patient, $s_1,\ldots,s_t = \underline{s}$. Interest is then centred on evaluating $P(D_i | \underline{S} = \underline{s})$ $i = 1,\ldots,m$.

It can be argued that disease causes symptoms and it is therefore more natural to consider $P(\underline{S} | D_i = d_i)$ and then apply Bayes theorem to give

$$P(D_i|\underline{S} = \underline{s}) = \frac{P(\underline{S}|D_i)P(D_i)}{\sum_{q=1}^{m} P(\underline{S}|D_q)P(D_q)} \qquad (2.1)$$

The random vector $\underline{S}$ comprises t indicants, so there will be at least 2^t possible indicant combinations $\underline{s}$. In general the available data set will be small in comparison to the number of indicant combinations, so direct estimation of $P(\underline{S}|D_i)$ is not feasible. However if we are able to assume that indicants are mutually independent within disease category, we have

$$P(\underline{S}|D_i) = \prod_{j=1}^{t} P(S_j|D_i) \qquad (2.2)$$

allowing us to compute indirect estimates using all the available cases.

The training data can be used to estimate the necessary probabilities as discussed in Crichton et al [2]. If our aim is to maximise the proportion of cases correctly classified then we should classify as HRC if

$$P(HRC|\underline{S}) \geq P(NHRC|\underline{S}) \qquad (2.3)$$

Using all 18 indicants and this classification rule, 85.1% of the training cases are correctly classified, the results are shown in table 1.

		Predict HRC	Predict NHRC	
True	HRC	50	25	75
True	NHRC	19	201	220
		69	226	295

Table 1 Classification of the training data using independent Bayes with 18 indicants.

The symptom probabilities were estimated from the training data, so it is more reasonable to judge the performance of the diagnostic system by considering the classification of the test data. The system correctly classifies 82.7% of the training cases, the classification results are shown in table 2.

	Predict HRC	Predict NHRC	
True HRC	16	8	24
True NHRC	15	94	109
	31	102	133

Table 2 Classification of the training data using independent Bayes with 18 indicants.

The assumption of mutual independence of indicants within disease category is central to this approach. This assumption has been greatly criticised in the literature and is certainly violated by this data set. However, it is difficult to explore the structure in the data set other than by considering the indicants pairwise since there are so few patients, particularly in the HRC category.

The effect of the incorrect assumption of independence is explored by Crichton et al [2] and by Hilden [7]; in general the consequence is over-confidence about the amount of evidence supporting a decision. Despite the lack of independence the method seems to perform reasonably well, however, knowledge of the stochastic structure would very likely permit exploitation of the symptom dependencies and lead to symptom redundancy.

Murray [11] explains that in discriminant analysis error rates do not increase monotonically with decreasing size of variable subset. A similar result can be demonstrated for the independent Bayes method [2]. If we wish to use a reduced set of indicants which subset should we use? A number of methods of variable selection are possible, for example the 'best combination' procedure suggested by Teather [13], a fully sequential procedure or a simple-step down procedure. The difficulties with the 'best combination' procedure are the choice of the number, say w, of the t indicants to consider and then the large amount of computation associated with considering all $\binom{t}{w}$ possible combinations. With sequential or stepwise procedures variables are considered one by one, so a pair of indicants that give perfect discrimination could be overlooked if neither of the two indicants are individually good discriminators.

All the suggested methods of variable selection have shortcomings. For illustrative purposes the simple step-down procedure is considered here. At any step, if there are v indicants remaining, the indicant for removal is that which leaves a set of (v - 1) indicants giving the highest proportion of correctly classified cases. Using this step-down approach with the chest pain data a problem is encountered at the first step. The maximum number of cases correctly classified using 17 indicants is 255, however there are two indicants we could drop which result in this number of correct classifications. How should we deal with such ties? It will matter which one we drop since this will influence the indicants dropped subsequently. A further problem is when to stop the step-down procedure. Initially the effect of dropping indicants is to slightly increase the number of cases correctly classified, so a possible rule might be to stop when the proportion correctly classified is less than when all indicants are used.

The stepwise procedure was carried out using the training data and two different tie rules were tried. The first rule removed the highest numbered contending indicant, the second rule removed the lowest numbered contender. The first rule suggested a set of 5 indicants, the second rule suggested a set of 6 indicants. Only three indicants were common to both sets. Applying the reduced indicant sets to the test data we obtain the results shown in table 3.

		Rule 1 (5 ind)		Rule 2 (6 ind)	
		Predict		Predict	
		HRC	NHRC	HRC	NHRC
	HRC	11	13	11	13
True	NHRC	8	101	9	100

Table 3 Classification results for the test data using independent Bayes and two different reduced sets of indicants.

Using step-down procedures there is a tendency for indicants with several categories to be retained. Some of the categories of such variables are uncommon and the associated probability estimates will be unreliable. It would be sensible to combine some categories of such variables, however, neither the step-down procedure nor consideration of pairs of indicants is able to provide the necessary structural information to enable us to combine categories whilst preserving the discriminatory power of the indicant.

To aid in the sensible selection of indicants it is clearly desirable to have some understanding of the inter-relationships between them. Given sufficient data one might consider a formal modelling approach to study the conditional independencies in the full crosstabulation of the data. However, with only 295 observations in the full table of over 500,000 cells this is clearly not a feasible strategy. Correspondence analysis provides a simple and quick exploratory method for representing these relationships, which can be used to suggest a restricted set of (unrelated) indicants for the application of the independent Bayes procedure.

3. CORRESPONDENCE ANALYSIS

The original idea underlying correspondence analysis dates back to Hirschfield [8] and was subsequently also suggested by Guttman [6]. The main development of correspondence analysis was in France under the inspiration of Benzécri and co-workers and has subsequently become a widely used technique for exploratory data analysis, in particular of survey data. A full account of the methods and their interpretation is given in Greenacre [5] and Lebart, Morineau and Warwick [10]. It is only recently that correspondence analysis has come to the attention of British statisticians who have begun to appreciate its uses (and limitations!). Its use will no doubt increase with the recent availability of english language software called SPAD.N by Lebart, Morineau and Lambert [9]. The IBM PC version of this software was used for all correspondence analyses presented in this paper.

3.1 Two-way Correspondence Analysis

The simplest form of correspondence analysis is that for a two-way table. The analysis consists of two principal component analyses; one is applied to the row profiles from the table using marginal row frequencies as weights and a χ^2-distance metric; the second is carried out in a similar fashion on the column profiles. These two principal component analyses are linked and allow the simultaneous display of the row and column categories on graphs of the principal axes taken two at a time.

Applying this technique to the 2 x 4 table of risk group by age for the training dataset gives a two-axis representation which explains 61% of the total variance and three-axis representation explaining 86%. Of itself this is of little interest as the full inter-relationship between age and risk group is given in the original table. However, it is possible to superimpose other variables on the principal axis plots. This gives a convenient method for screening important indicants which may be related to risk group (which is of direct interest here) and also to age. Each category of these supplementary variables is plotted at the centre of gravity of the responses on the age x risk group categories, with some axis dependent rescaling. A test value can be obtained for each co-ordinate of each supplementary variable category. This test statistic has expected value zero under the null hypothesis that the individuals in a particular category are chosen at random from the set of all individuals. Large absolute values (>2) of this test statistic indicate a possible relationship between the category and the axis. Figure 1 shows a plot of the first two principal axes along with potentially important supplementary categories.

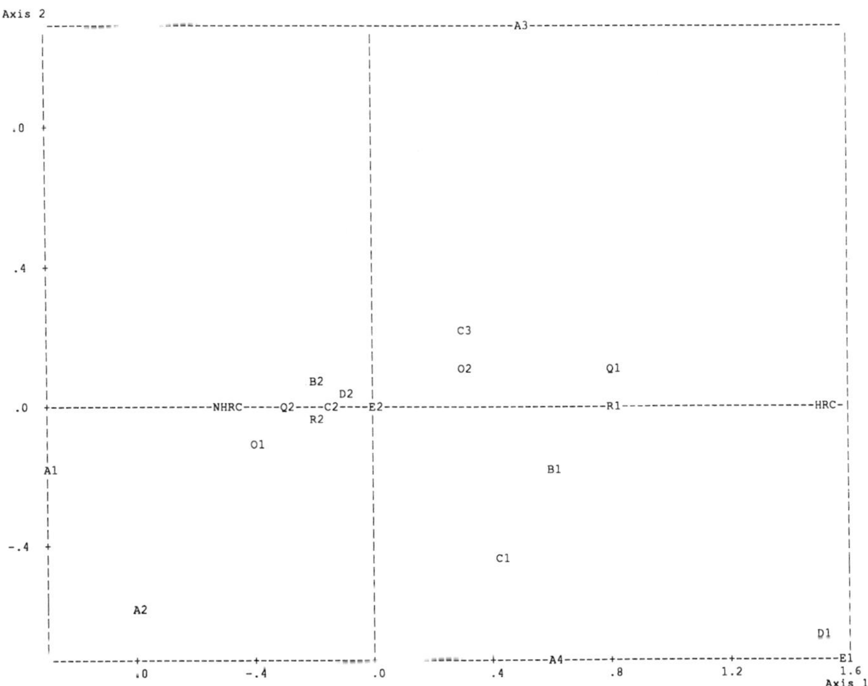

Fig. 1 First two axes of correspondence analysis of risk group by age with supplementary variables

This suggests the importance of history of myocardial infarction (M.I.) [variable R], history of angina [variable Q], worse on coughing [variable O], looking very ill [variable D] and clinical shock [variable E]. We also see the close association between some of these indicants, notably looking very ill [D] and clinical shock [E], and also a history of M.I. [R] or angina [Q]; their closeness on the plot indicates that they have similar age x risk group profiles.

3.2 Multiple Correspondence Analysis

While the above analysis is informative in terms of predictors of risk group, the selection of risk group by age as the table to study is somewhat arbitrary. A more natural analysis is to consider the association between the 18 indicants and then to attempt to relate any structure there to the risk groups. This can be achieved using multiple correspondence analysis which is a simple extension of the correspondence analysis of a two-way table. Writing Z as the (295 x $\Sigma_{i=1}^{18}$ (no. categories for indicant i)) incidence matrix of the indicant categories, a multiple correspondence analysis is a simple correspondence analysis of Z^TZ. The matrix Z^TZ is usually referred to as the 'Burt matrix' and is simply the symmetric matrix of all pairwise marginal tables, and is analogous to the covariance matrix for continuous variables. Clearly any analysis based on this can only take account of first-order interactions.

From the correspondence analysis we can again obtain plots of the categories on graphs of the principal axes, along with measures of the contribution of each indicant to any particular axis and the explanation of each category by each axis. This allows us to interpret the axes in terms of the important indicants and categories and suggests which indicants or categories may be closely related. Of particular interest here is the display of risk group as a supplementary variable, see figure 2, where we see that the first axis is strongly associated with risk group. Looking at the indicants we again see that the history of M.I. [R] and angina [Q] are closely related as also are looking ill [D], clinical shock [E] and visible sweat [F]. It is also clear that with respect to risk group categories 1 and 2 of age [A] are closely related as also are categories 2,4 and 5 of the site indicant [H].

Instead of summarising the patients by the two risk groups it is possible to plot each individual, see figure 3. This gives a clear picture of why it may be that some cases are very easily correctly diagnosed whereas others are much more difficult.

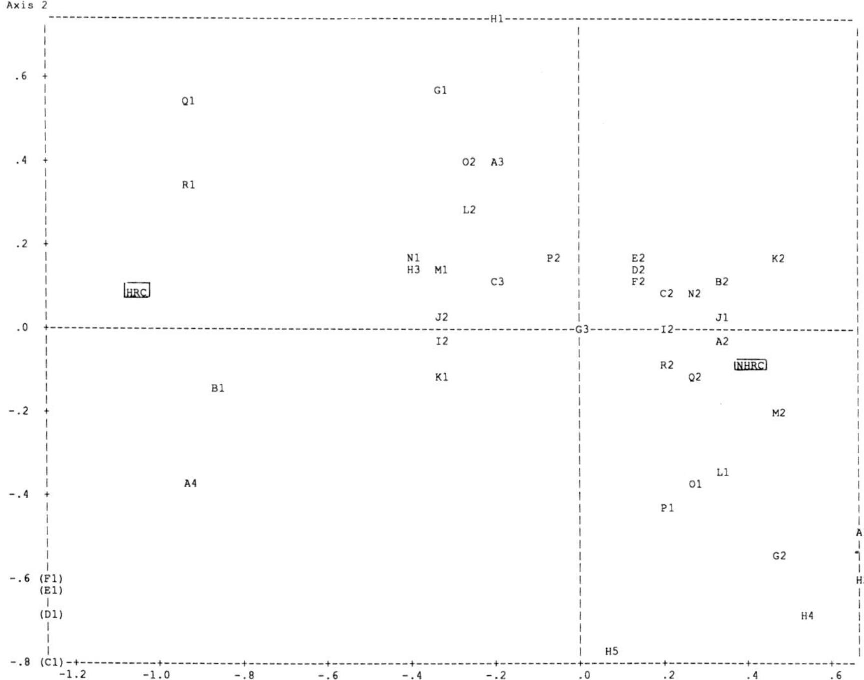

Fig. 2 First two principal axes of multiple correspondence analysis of 18 indicants

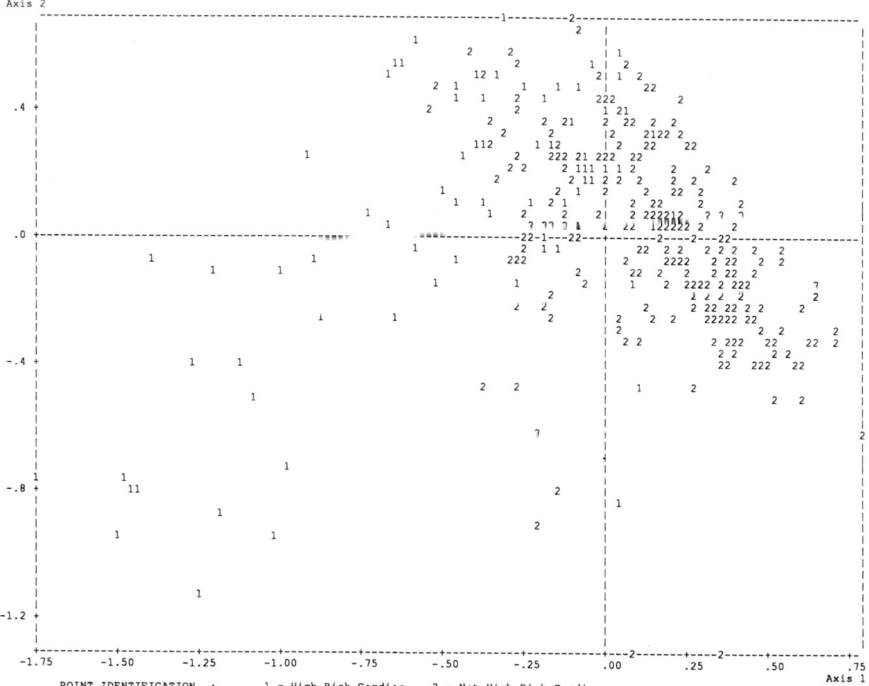

Fig. 3 Plot of individuals for training dataset

In a similar fashion we can plot the 133 individuals from the test dataset, see figure 4. This shows a similar pattern to that for the training data, but with fewer clearly defined high risk cardiac cases.

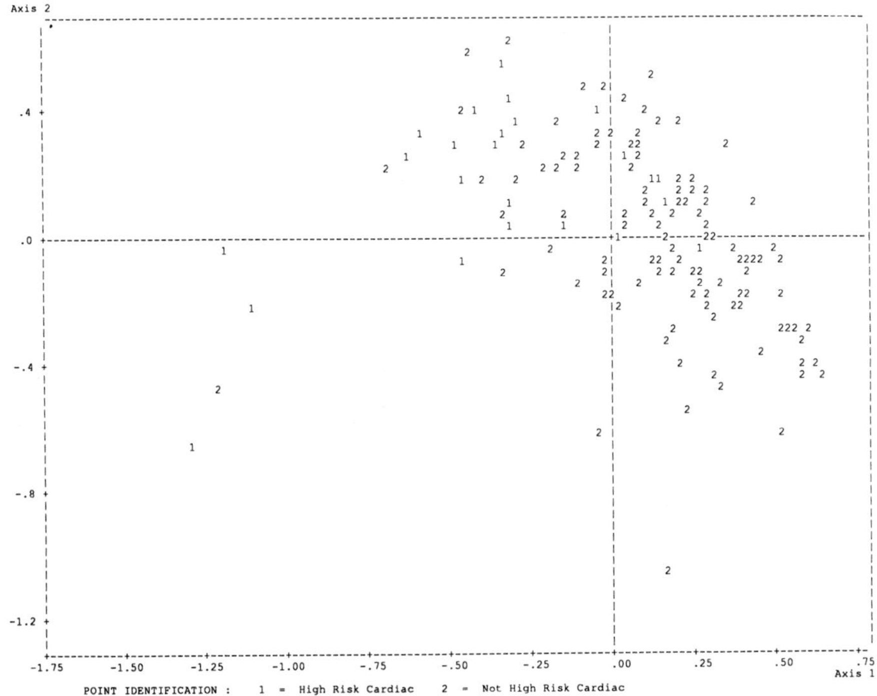

Fig. 4 Plot of individuals for test dataset

The plots presented here have focused solely on the first two principal axes, many other plots are of course possible, although none give any particularly clear picture. The strong association of axis 1 with risk group makes it of particular interest.

From Figure 2 it can be seen that the indicant categories A4, B1, C1, D1, E1, F1, H3, Q1 and R1 are located close to HRC whilst another category of each of these indicants is located closer to NHRC than to HRC. This suggests that these might be good indicants to include in the independent Bayes decision system. However it is also clear from figure 2 that indicants D,E,F are closely related, thus in order to comply with the independence assumption only one should be included in the Bayes system. Similarly only one of Q and R should be included.

Considering the contribution measure provided by SPAD.N, looks very ill [D] was selected from D,E,F. Similarly history of M.I. [R] was selected from Q and R. Thus the variables suggested for use in the independent Bayes system are age (in 3 groups) [A], arrival by ambulance [B], diastolic blood pressure [C], looks very ill [D], site of pain (in 3 groups) [H] and history of M.I. [R].

Applying the independent Bayes method using these six indicants we correctly classify 85.4% of the training cases, making correct classifications for 44 HRC cases and 208 NHRC cases. The classification of the test data results in 88.7% of the decisions being correct, the results are shown in table 4.

	Predict HRC	Predict NHRC	
HRC	12	12	24
True NHRC	3	106	109
	15	118	133

Table 4 Classification of the test data using independent Bayes and the indicants suggested by the correspondence analysis.

The results compare favourably with those from the previous section.

4. DISCUSSION

The results of this analysis show the potential value of correspondence analysis as a tool for identifying and exploiting the structure in a set of clinical data. As with many exploratory methods there is no formal 'test' of whether or not an indicant should be included. However, a decision to include based upon subjective impressions from the plot, which shows the relationship to the other variables, is seen to be at least as good as making judgements on the basis of changes of 1 or 2 in the number of correct classifications (the pseudo-test used in the step-down procedure).

It is clear from the figures that there are likely to be several subsets of the indicants of similar discriminatory power. It is therefore unreasonable to necessarily expect to identify the 'best indicant subset.

The approach using correspondence analysis can be simply generalised to deal with problems with a larger number of diagnostic groups. However, in practice, it may be more difficult to identify useful general discriminatory indicants, particularly if most are binary, since they will tend to be associated with a particular diagnosis. It may be valuable to investigate a multiple decision problem as a series of binary problems.

In the proposed independent Bayes system all six indicants are given equal weight. Whilst there is no obvious reason why any other weighting system should be used for this example, one can envisage situations in which unequal weights might be desirable, or where weighted combinations of related indicants might be preferable to selecting a single representative indicant. Further work is necessary to investigate whether correspondence analysis could provide a sensible weighting strategy for the indicants, perhaps related to their distance from the diagnostic categories or from the first axis.

A naive approach has been taken to the decision problem in this paper. Firstly, it is unrealistic to be interested in maximising the proportion of correctly classified cases since the errors are not equally bad. This could be dealt with by introducing a utility structure into the independent Bayes system as described in Crichton et al [2]. It is also unrealistic to make decisions with a strict probability cut point at 0.5, particularly as no account has been taken of the possibly large variances associated with the probability estimates. In practice, if the probability of HRC was very high, say greater than 0.8, or was very low, say less than 0.2, the decision to admit to CCU or not might be made immediately; otherwise more information would be collected or further tests done.

REFERENCES

[1] Adams, I.D. et al., (1986) Computer aided diagnosis of acute abdominal pain: a multicentre study. *Br. Med. J.*, **293**, 800-804.

[2] Crichton, N.J., Fryer, J.G. and Spicer, C.G., (1987) Some points on the use of independent Bayes to diagnose acute abdominal pain. *Stats. in Medicine*, **6**, 945-959.

[3] de Dombal, F.T., Leaper, D.J., Staniland, J.R., McCann, A. and Horrocks, J., (1972) Computer aided diagnosis of acute abdominal pain. *Br. Med. J.*, **2**, 9-13.

[4] du Boulay, G.H., Teather, D., Harling, D. and Clarke, G., (1977) Improvements in computer-assisted diagnosis of cerebral tumours. *Br. J. of Radiology,* **50**, 849-854.

[5] Greenacre, M.J., (1984) Theory and applications of correspondence analysis, Academic Press, London.

[6] Guttman, L., (1941) 'The quantification of a class of attributes' in The Prediction of Personal Adjustment, P. Horst et al., Editors, Social Science Research Council, New York.

[7] Hilden, J., (1984) Statistical diagnosis based on conditional independence does not require it. *Computers in Biology and Medicine,* **14**, 429-435.

[8] Hirschfield, H.O., (1935) A connection between correlation and contingency. *Camb. Phil. Soc. Proc. (Math. Proc.),* **31**, 520-524.

[9] Lebart, L., Morineau, A. and Lambert, T., SPAD.N.: Statistical package for the analysis of data, CISIA, Sèvres.

[10] Lebart, L., Morineau, A. and Warwick, K.M., (1984) Multivariate descriptive statistical analysis, Wiley, New York.

[11] Murray, G.D., (1977) A cautionary note on selection of variables in discriminant analysis. *Applied Stats.* **26**, 246-250.

[12] Spiegelhalter, D.J. and Knill-Jones, R.P., (1984) Statistical and knowledge-based approaches to clinical decision support systems, with an application in gastreoenterology. *J.R. Statist. Soc. A,* **147**, 35-76.

[13] Teather, D., (1974) Statistical techniques for diagnosis. *J.R. Statist. Soc. A,* **137**, 231 244.

[14] Titterington, D.M. et al., (1981) Comparison of discrimination techniques applied to a complex data set of head injured patients. *J.R. Statist. Soc. A,* **144**, 145-174.

ACKNOWLEDGEMENT

We are grateful to Dr. P.A. Emerson and his co-workers at the Westminster Hospital for allowing us access to part of their dataset.

INTERPRETATION OF ORAL GLUCOSE TOLERANCE TEST RESULTS

M. Farrow and A.H. Leyland
(Department of Mathematics and Computer Studies, Sunderland Polytechnic, Priestman Building, Green Terrace, Sunderland)

ABSTRACT

The oral glucose tolerance test is used, for example, to help in deciding whether a diabetic patient should be considered insulin dependent. The glucose concentrations in blood samples, taken before oral administration of glucose and at intervals thereafter, are measured. It is also possible to determine the concentration, in the blood samples, of C-peptide, which is thought to be a useful indicator of insulin production.

In this paper we consider the measurement of response using both glucose and C-peptide data. An approach using a general multivariate normal model for the data vector is compared with a curve fitting approach using exponentially damped polynomials and allowing for between - subject variation by means of a two-stage model. In this latter approach the group parameter estimates are determined via the E.M. algorithm.

1. INTRODUCTION

This paper is concerned with an attempt to help clinicians in the interpretation of data which might be used to help determine the appropriate treatment for elderly diabetics. Depending on the severity of the disease and on how well it is being controlled, these patients may be treated by a special diet, by a combination of diet and drugs or by insulin. Clearly it is important that those patients who need insulin should be given it. It is also highly desirable that those who do not need insulin should not receive it. As time passes, patients may become insulin dependent. Some patients may also cease to be insulin dependent if the control of their disease is improved.

The decision whether or not a patient should be given insulin involves consideration of many factors, not all of which are directly related to the severity of the disease. In this paper we are concerned only with measurement of the severity of the disease.

One tool which is used to measure severity of diabetes is the oral glucose tolerance test (O.G.T.T.). After a period without food patients are given glucose orally. Blood samples are taken immediately before the glucose is given and at intervals thereafter. The concentration of glucose in each sample is determined and, roughly speaking, the quicker the glucose concentration returns to its fasting level the more healthy is the patient.

The study with which we are concerned involved two new features. One was the belief of the experimenters that methods of analysis of O.G.T.T. results designed for young patients may need to be altered to suit the elderly because of a generally slower response rate in old people. The other was the determination, not only of glucose concentration, but also of C-peptide concentration in the blood samples. The concentration of C-peptide is believed to indicate insulin production.

Seventy five subjects, in five groups of fifteen each, were given O.G.T.T.s. Group 1 consisted of elderly people who were not diabetic. Groups 2 and 3 consisted of elderly diabetics who were not being treated with insulin. Those in Group 2 were considered to be "poorly controlled" while those in Group 3 were described as "well controlled". Group 4 contained elderly insulin dependent diabetics. Group 5 contained young people who were not diabetic. Blood samples were taken immediately before the glucose was given and then after 30, 60, 90 and 120 minutes. Typical responses from each of the five groups are shown in Figure 1. The experiment and its medical background are described by Wickramasinghe et al. [1].

A number of authors have proposed indices of severity of diabetes based on the glucose concentrations from O.G.T.T.s. Ackerman, Rosevear and McGuckin [2] suggested that the blood glucose concentration would follow a damped sinusoid and that the period of the corresponding undamped wave could be used to measure diabetes. Healthy people would have short periods and diabetics would have longer periods. In the 1960's the difficulty of fitting such curves to data by non linear regression prevented the use of this method. In the 1980's the availability of microcomputers could remove this obstacle. Billewicz, Anderson and Lind [3] proposed an index which involves the time to peak blood glucose concentration and an approximation of the area under the curve and above the fasting level. This method proved impossible to use with the data considered here because of the lack, in many cases, of a clear peak within the timespan covered by the data. In [1] the increase over one hour in C-peptide concentration divided by the corresponding increase in glucose concentration, used in combination with fasting blood glucose concentration appears to give reasonably good separation of the groups. This is illustrated in Figure 2.

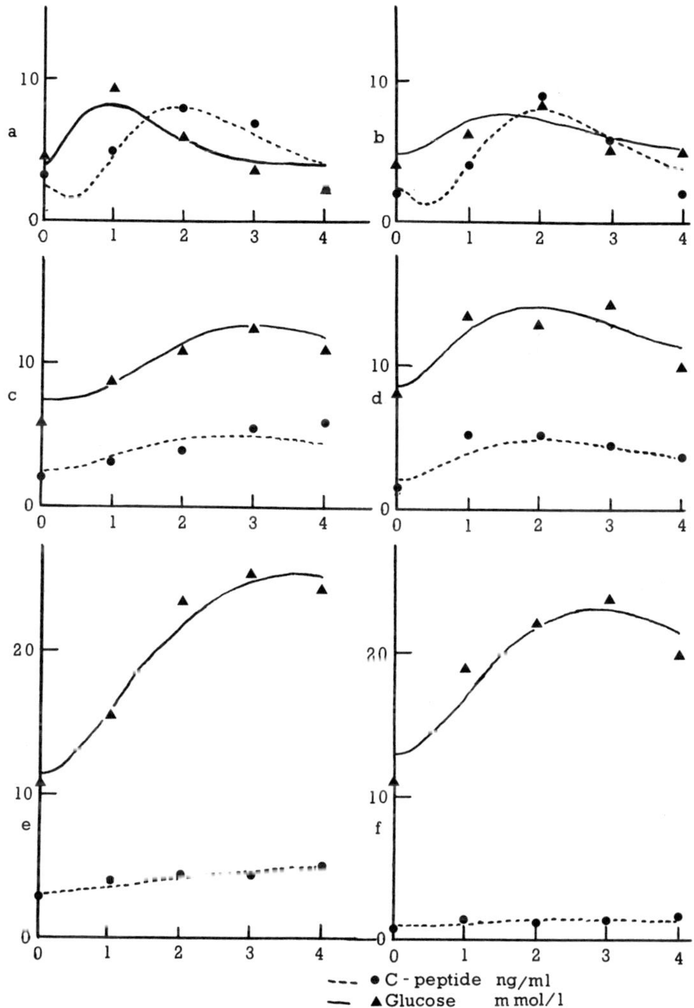

Fig. 1 Typical data with fitted curves: a,b Group 1, c,d Group 3, e Group 2, f Group 4.

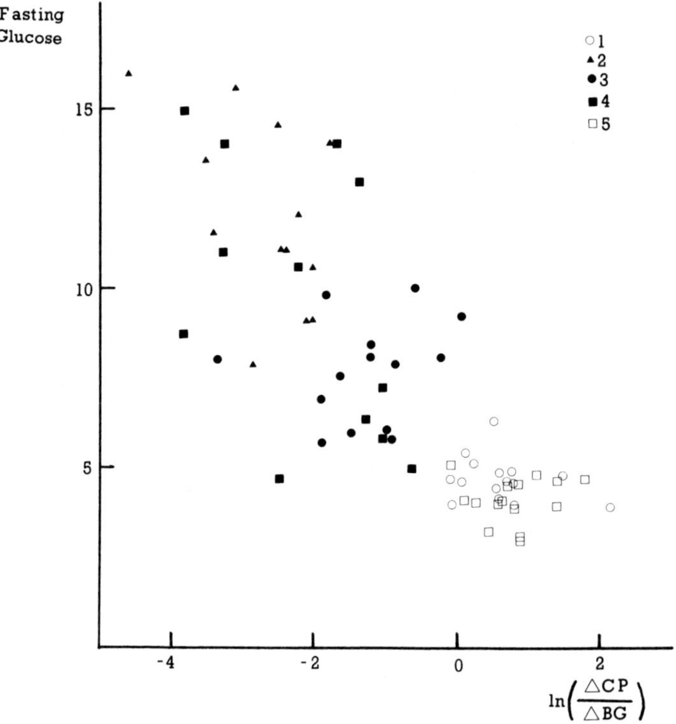

Fig. 2 Log. of one hour increment in C-peptide divided by one hour increment in glucose against initial glucose observation.

In Section 3 below a curve fitting approach is described. As will be seen, the approach is somewhat different to that of Ackerman et al. and involves the C-peptide values as well as the glucose concentration. This is compared with a more straightforward multivariate analysis which is described in Section 2.

The data also include the body mass index which is thought to be useful in determining insulin dependence. This has not been used in this paper because here we are particularly interested in comparing methods of analysing the short time series and measuring the biological response to a stimulus. Further work on the clinical application should include consideration of the body mass index.

2. MULTIVARIATE APPROACH

In this section we treat the glucose and C-peptide measurements on a single patient as forming a multivariate observation $\underline{y} = (y_1,\ldots,y_{10})'$ where $y_1,\ldots, y_5$ are the C-peptide measurements in order and $y_6,\ldots,y_{10}$ are the corresponding glucose measurements. Either these data, or their logarithms, will be considered to be taken from multivariate normal distributions, one distribution for each group. A Bayesian approach is used. The results on Bayesian inference for multivariate normal distributions used in this section are based on [4].

Suppose we make n independent observations on a multivariate normal distribution with k variables, mean vector $\underline{M}$ and precision matrix R. In this case n = 15 and k = 10. Suppose our prior distribution for $\underline{M}$ and R is as follows. Given that R = r, $\underline{M}$ has a multivariate normal distribution with mean $\underline{\mu}$ and precision matrix νr, where $\nu>0$. The marginal prior for R is a Wishart distribution with $\alpha>k-1$ degrees of freedom and precision matrix τ. Then the posterior distribution of $\underline{M}$ and R is as follows. Given that R = r, $\underline{M}$ has a multivariate normal distribution with mean $\underline{\mu}^*$ and precision matrix $(\nu+n)r$ where

$$\underline{\mu}^* = \frac{\nu\underline{\mu}+n\bar{\underline{y}}}{\nu+n}$$

and $\bar{\underline{y}}$ is the sample mean vector. The marginal distribution of R is Wishart with $\alpha+n$ degrees of freedom and precision matrix τ^* where

$$\tau^* = \tau+s+\frac{\nu n}{\nu+n}(\underline{\mu}-\bar{\underline{y}})(\underline{\mu}-\bar{\underline{y}})'$$

and

$$s = \sum_{i=1}^{n}(\underline{y}_i-\bar{\underline{y}})(\underline{y}_i-\bar{\underline{y}})'$$

Now suppose we intend to make a new observation $\underline{y}^+$. The joint distribution of $\underline{y}^+$ and R is as follows. Given that R = r, $\underline{y}^+$ has a multivariate normal distribution with mean $\underline{\mu}^*$ and precision matrix

$$\frac{\nu+n}{\nu+n+1} r.$$

The marginal distribution of R is its posterior marginal as before. Thus the marginal predictive distribution for $\underline{y}^+$ is multivariate t with $\alpha+n-k+1$ degrees of freedom, location vector $\underline{\mu}^*$ and precision matrix

$$\frac{\nu+n}{\nu+n+1}(\alpha+n-k+1)\,\tau^{*-1}$$

Let the probability density function of this predictive distribution be $f_j(\underline{y}^+)$, $j=1,..,5$. Let the prior probability that a new individual belongs to group j be p_j. Then the posterior probability is

$$\frac{p_j f_j(\underline{y}^+)}{\sum_{k=1}^{5} p_k f_k(\underline{y}^+)}$$

and the ratio of posterior probabilities for groups j and k is simply

$$\frac{p_j f_j(\underline{y}^+)}{p_k f_k(\underline{y}^+)}.$$

It is not our aim at this stage to provide posterior probabilities, particularly since the allocation of patients to groups in the first place is certainly not beyond question and each of the Groups 2, 3 and 4 contains patients with a range of severities of diabetes. However ratios such as $f_1(\underline{y})/f_4(\underline{y})$ might provide useful indicators.

While a proper prior is clearly to be preferred in practice, in order to avoid prejudicing the comparison with the methods of Section 3 we will now use the improper prior obtained by letting $\nu\to 0$, $\alpha\to -1$ and τ tend to a matrix of zeros, ([4] p. 197). This leads to a predictive distribution for $\underline{y}^+$ which is multivariate t with n-k degrees of freedom,

location vector $\underline{\bar{y}}$ and precision matrix

$$\frac{n(n-k)}{n+1}S^{-1}.$$

We can write the probability density function as

$$m_{n,k} = [\,1+\frac{n}{n+1}g(y^+)]^{-n/2}|S|^{-1/2}$$

where

$$m_{n,k} = \frac{\Gamma(\frac{n}{2})\,(\frac{n}{n+1})^{k/2}}{\Gamma(\frac{n-k}{2})\,\pi^{k/2}}$$

depends only on n and k and $g(\underline{y}^+) = (\underline{y}^+-\underline{\bar{y}})'S^{-1}(\underline{y}^+-\underline{\bar{y}})$. Using the subscript in an obvious way to denote the group to which the statistics refer and writing $g_j(\underline{y}^+) = (\underline{y}^+-\underline{\bar{y}}_j)'S_j^{-1}(\underline{y}^+-\underline{\bar{y}}_j)$, the ratio $f_j(\underline{y}^+)/f_k(\underline{y}^+)$ becomes

$$\left[\frac{1+\frac{n}{n+1}g_j(\underline{y}^+)}{1+\frac{n}{n+1}g_k(\underline{y}^+)}\right]^{-n/2}\left[\frac{|S_j|}{|S_k|}\right]^{-1/2}$$

for two groups of equal size. Thus the posterior probabilities would depend on the quadratic forms $g(\underline{y}^+)$.

Writing $h_j(\underline{y}^+) = \ln[\,1+\frac{n}{n+1}g_j(y^+)]$ we obtain

$$\ln\left\{\frac{f_j(\underline{y}^+)}{f_k(\underline{y}^+)}\right\} = \frac{1}{2}\{\ln|S_j|-\ln|S_k|+n[\,h_j(\underline{y}^+)-h_k(\underline{y}^+)]\}$$

Plots of $h_j(\underline{y}^+)$ against $h_k(\underline{y}^+)$ have been found effective in showing the separation of the groups. While it would be possible to plot the values of the probability density functions rather than $h(\underline{y}^+)$, this seems unnecessary since we are merely looking for a concise numerical description of a patient's condition. It should be noted, of course, that the points plotted include the groups which were used to determine the coefficients.

Figure 3 shows $h_1(\underline{y})$ (elderly controls) plotted against $h_4(\underline{y})$ (insulin). It can be seen that the controls and insulin dependent patients are well separated and that the non-insulin dependent diabetics generally fall between these groups.

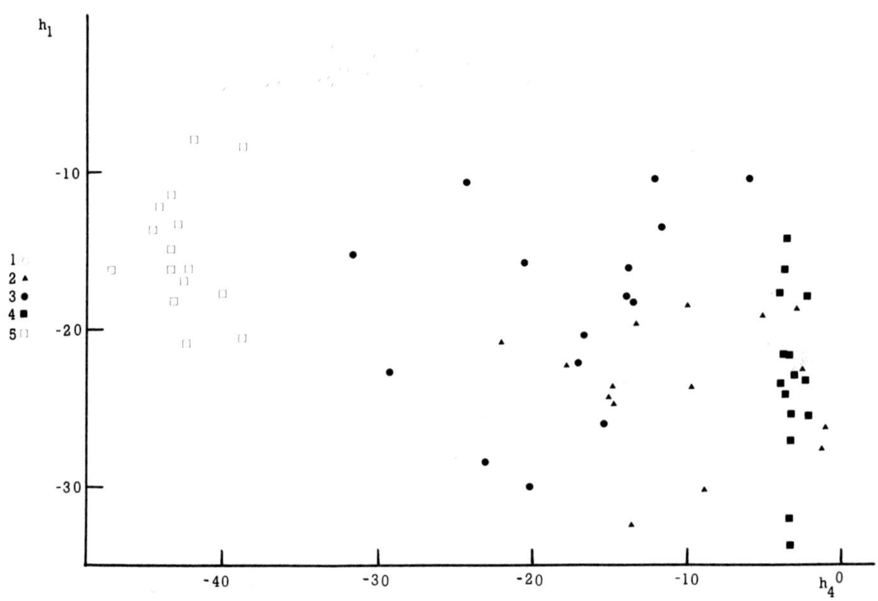

Fig. 3 h_1 against h_4 (raw data)

However, it has to be conceded that the separation certainly appears to be no better than that obtained by the simpler method of [1]. On the other hand it should be remembered that Groups 2, 3 and 4 contained patients with varying degrees of illness. In fact after the data were collected, but before the C-peptide values were available, several patients were given changes of treatment on other grounds. Four patients were taken off insulin. These turn out to be the four members of Group 4 with the smallest $h_4(\underline{y})$ values. Eight patients in Group 2 (poorly controlled) were put on insulin. These turn out to include the five with the greatest values of $h_4(\underline{y})-h_1(\underline{y})$.

Figure 4 is the same as Figure 3 except that the data were transformed by taking logs. This appears to have improved the results. This time the four patients taken off insulin were the four with the greatest values of $h_1(\underline{y})$ in Group 4. The eight patients started on insulin include the six members of Group 2 with the smallest values of $h_1(\underline{y})$.

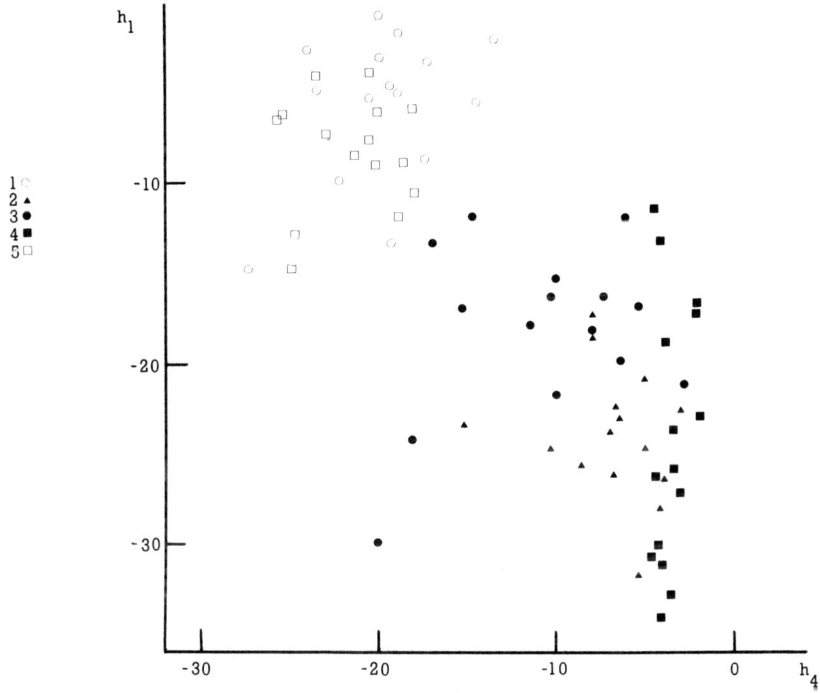

Fig. 4 h_1 against h_4 (logarithmically transformed data)

Consideration of $h_2(\underline{y})$ and $h_3(\underline{y})$ does not appear to contribute much to the ability to predict the changes in treatment which were made.

It would appear that $h_1(\underline{y})$, calculated using the logs of the data, is the most useful of the measures considered here. However, in order to avoid mistakenly classifying, for example, a healthy person with a response like that of a young person as ill because the response is atypical, it is perhaps better to consider $h_4(\underline{y})$ as well.

It might be thought that a more direct approach, as follows, might be preferable. Suppose the mean vector for healthy elderly patients is $\underline{\mu}_H$ and that there exists a mean vector $\underline{\mu}_I$ for strongly insulin dependent patients. Then we might suppose that there is a value λ_i for each patient so that that patient has a "mean" vector $\lambda_i\underline{\mu}_H+(1-\lambda i)\underline{\mu}_I$. Given a suitable prior for λ_i we should be able to estimate $\underline{\mu}_H$ and $\underline{\mu}_I$ and then obtain values for the individual λ_is. Unfortunately an attempt at this method led to very disappointing results.

3. CURVE FITTING APPROACH

The method described in Section 2 did not exploit any beliefs we might have about the form the graphs of C-peptide and glucose against time might take. In this section we consider fitting curves of a specific type to the data. Some of the "parameters" of these curves are allowed to vary between individuals within a group but these "parameters" are then themselves considered to take the form of a random sample for each patient from some underlying distribution for the group. The problem is then to estimate the parameters of these group distributions and then find posterior expectations etc. of individuals' curve parameters in the hope that these might be useful indicators of the condition of patients.

Two stage models like this, where regression parameters for an individual are considered to be random samples from an underlying distribution, have been used by a number of authors, for example Laird and Ware [5]. The main difference here is in the use of a nonlinear regression.

The obvious form of curve to try is the damped sinusoid suggested in [2]. Both C-peptide and glucose would be expected to follow damped sinusoids with the same period and damping but out of phase. However, it quickly became apparent that we would not get good results with such curves. This may be because of the shortness of our series, showing no signs of having reached maxima and certainly no signs of periodicity or damping.

Instead we have adopted exponentially damped polynomials. This class of curves was proposed for a related application by Crowder and Tredger [6]. Suppose the C-peptide value at time t after administration of glucose is p(t). Then we write

$$p(t) = \alpha_o+e^{-\Theta t}\alpha(t)$$

where $\alpha(t)$ is a polynomial in t. The constant in $\alpha(t)$ was set to zero so that the C-peptide concentration would return to its fasting level as $t\to\infty$. The coefficient of t in $\alpha(t)$ was also set to zero so that the first derivative would initially be zero. Polynomials of degree three and four were tried. There appeared to be little, if any, advantage in using quartics when compared to cubics. Use of a quadratic would not allow the time to reach the peak concentration to vary for fixed Θ. For these reasons in what follows we assume

$$p(t) = \alpha_0+e^{-\Theta t}\{\alpha_2 t^2+\alpha_3 t^3\}.$$

Similarly, for the glucose concentration, we write

$$g(t) = \beta_0+e^{-\Theta t}\{\beta_2 t^2+\beta_3 t^3\}.$$

We assumed independent additive normal errors so that the observations at time t, t = 0,1,2,3,4, are

$$p_t = p(t)+\varepsilon_{pt}, \quad \varepsilon_{pt}\sim \text{i.i.d.}N(0,\sigma_p^2)$$

$$g_t = g(t)+\varepsilon_{gt}, \quad \varepsilon_{gt}\sim \text{i.i.d.}N(0,\sigma_g^2)$$

We did not allow Θ to vary between the individuals in a group, although it varies between groups. This is partly in order to simplify the calculations but also because, with so few observations per series, we felt that allowing individual values of Θ might, in a sense, overparameterise the model. We are working on other applications where similar non linear parameters are given between-individual distributions. Crowder [7] used a gamma distribution for the between individual variation of Θ. We give the six α and β parameters a multivariate normal distribution

A full Bayesian analysis of this model would make great computational demands simply because of the large number of parameters, especially variances and covariances. However, the maximum likelihood estimates of the group parameters can be found relatively easily via an E.M. algorithm and so we have used these as an approximation to the posterior mode for vague prior information.

The algorithm we have used is based on that described by Dempster, Rubin and Tsutakawa [8]. Our algorithm differs in two main respects from that of [8]. Firstly we have two error variances σ_p^2 and σ_g^2 and secondly we have the non linear parameter Θ. We could deal with Θ in either of two ways. We could maximise the "complete data" likelihood with respect to Θ simultaneously with the other group parameters at each M stage. Alternatively we could leave Θ fixed until the E.M. algorithm converges then start the E.M. algorithm again with a new value of Θ and thus search for the value of Θ which maximises the likelihood with all the other parameters set at their conditional maximum likelihood values given Θ. For reasons of computational convenience we actually used the latter approach.

Figure 1 shows some typical fitted curves, that is curves obtained using the maximum likelihood estimates of the group parameters and the expectations of the α and β parameters given the individual's data and treating the group parameters as known. Closer fits are, of course, obtained if quartics rather than cubics are used. In some cases a local minimum occurs in the fitted C-peptide curve before the maximum.

Using the maximum likelihood estimates of the group parameters and using the estimated group means for the α and β parameters leads to the curves shown in Figure 5. Two versions of the curves for Group 4 are given. The second version was obtained by omitting the four patients who were subsequently taken off insulin from all of the calculations. This has little effect on the shapes of the curves but alters the levels.

Writing the model for an individual patient as

$$\underline{y} = X_\Theta \underline{b} + \underline{\varepsilon}$$

where X_Θ is a 10x8 matrix whose elements depend on Θ, $\underline{b}$ is multivariate normal with mean $\underline{\mu}$ and dispersion matrix V_b and $\underline{\varepsilon}$ is multivariate normal with zero mean and dispersion matrix V_ε, we obtain the probability density function for $\underline{y}$ as

$$(2\pi)^{-5} |V_y|^{-\frac{1}{2}} \exp\{-\tfrac{1}{2}(\underline{y}-\underline{\mu})' V_y^{-1} (\underline{y}-\underline{\mu})\}$$

where

$$V_y = X_\Theta V_b X_\Theta' + V_\varepsilon$$

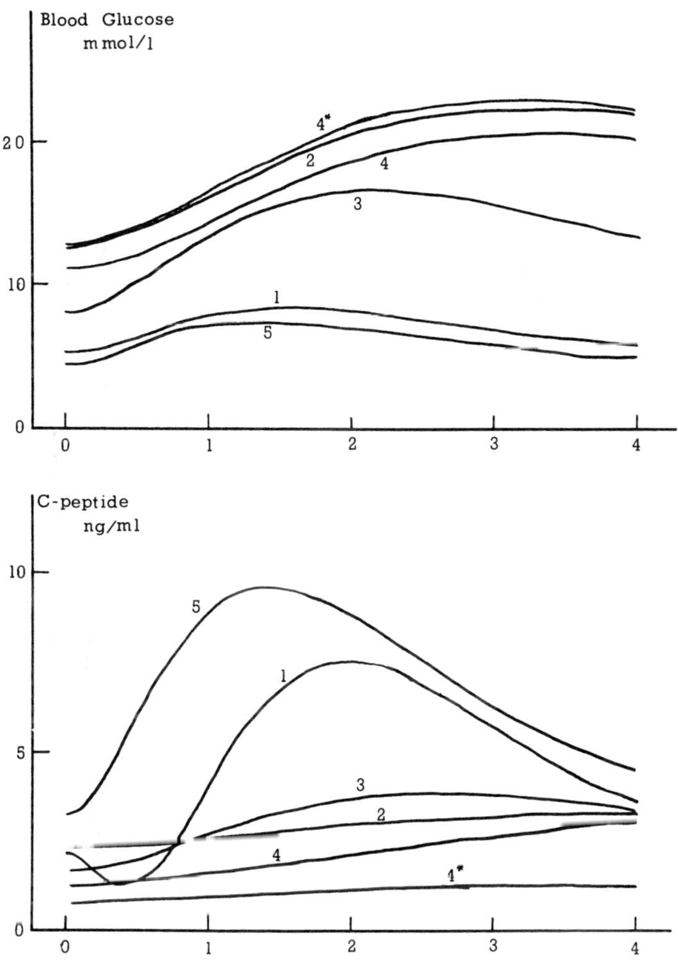

Fig. 5 Mean curves for groups (4*: Group 4 with patients transferred out omitted).

Let $k_j(\underline{y})$ be this function evaluated with the parameters set equal to their maximum likelihood estimates in Group j.

For each individual we can evaluate $k_j(\underline{y})$ for each j and by choosing the group which gives the largest value we can obtain a rough idea of the discriminations between the groups. For this purpose the four patients in Group 4 who were taken off insulin were omitted from the estimation. Using this method, fourteen of the seventy five subjects were allocated to groups other than their own. These fourteen included the four in Group 4 who were, in fact, taken off insulin. All of these were allocated to Group 3 (well controlled) which is, in fact, what happened in practice. Two other members of Group 4 were allocated, by a very narrow margin, to Group 2 (poorly controlled). Six patients in Group 2 were allocated to Group 4 (insulin). In fact four of these six and four others were subsequently given insulin. Two patients in Group 3 were also allocated to Group 4. In most cases where the actual treatment changes differed from the reallocations by this method the difference between $k(\underline{y})$ for the actual group, after treatment changes, and the minimum value of $k_j(\underline{y})$ for the subject was small.

The integral of excess glucose above the fasting level may be calculated as

$$I_g = \int_0^\infty g(t)-\beta_0 . dt = \theta^{-4}(2\beta_2\theta+6\beta_3).$$

Similarly

$$I_p = \int_0^\infty p(t)-\alpha_0 . dt = \theta^{-4}(2\alpha_2\theta+6\alpha_3).$$

The posterior expectations of these quantities, using Group 1 estimates for the group parameters, may be calculated easily. Writing these posterior expectations as

$$\hat{I}_g = \underline{m}_g{}'y+c_g$$

and

$$\hat{I}_p = \underline{m}'_p y+c_p$$

we obtain

$\underline{m}_g{}' = (-0.02, -0.07, -0.08, -0.05, -0.03, 0.00, 0.03, 0.08, 0.05, 0.02)$

and

$$\underline{m}_p' = (-0.02, 0.09, 0.16, 0.09, 0.03, -0.03, -0.09, -0.04, -0.02, -0.02)$$

Notice how the observations after one hour appear to be particularly important. The results are shown in Figure 6 where the values plotted are the differences from the Group 1 mean. It will be seen that the healthier patients generally have smaller glucose excesses and greater C-peptide excesses. The four members of Group 4 with the greatest C-peptide excesses in that group are the four who were subsequently taken off insulin.

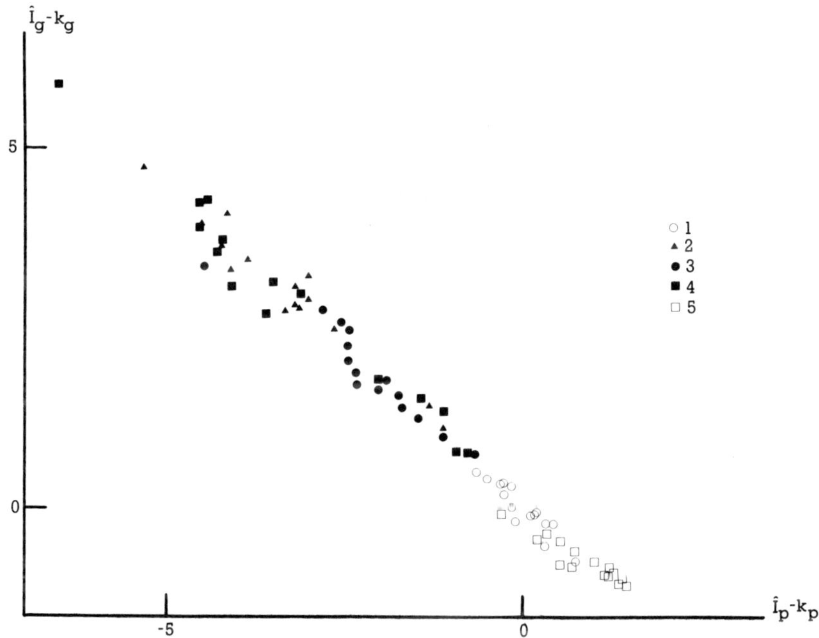

Fig. 6 Estimated integrals of excess C-peptide ($\hat{I}_p$) and glucose ($\hat{I}_g$), using Group 1 parameters (differences from Group 1 means).

A comparison with the results of [1] is provided in Figure 7 in which $\ln(\hat{I}_p/\hat{I}_g)$ is plotted against the posterior expectation of fasting glucose concentration (using Group 1 estimates for the group parameters).

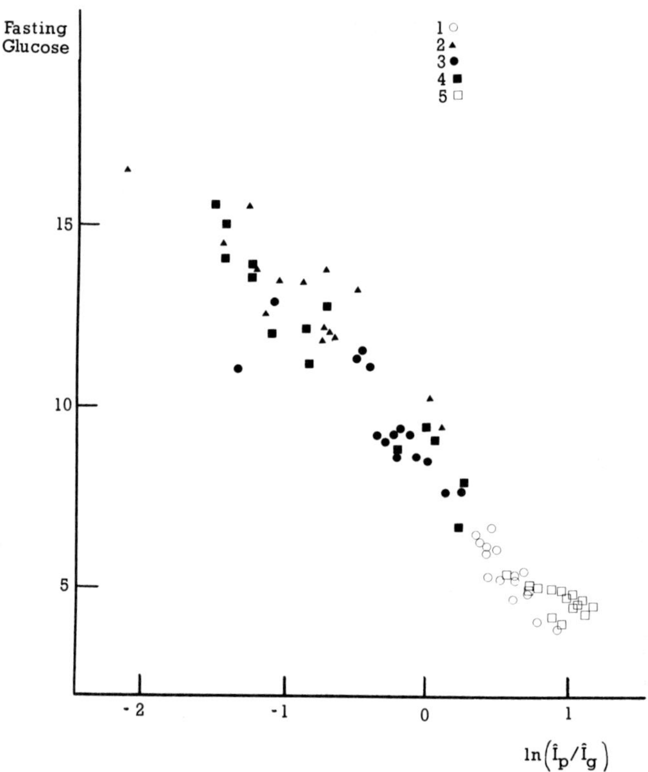

Fig. 7 Log. of estimated C-peptide integral divided by estimated glucose integral against estimated fasting glucose (using Group 1 parameters).

4. DISCUSSION

The comparison of the different approaches to the analysis of the data described here, or indeed comparison with the simpler method of [1], does not lead to firm conclusions.

Further work is needed on the curve fitting approach, particularly to investigate the many different quantities which could be calculated in order to try to obtain a one or two-dimensional summary of a patient's response. It should also be remembered that the samples used here were small.

However, it can be said in favour of the curve fitting approach that, assuming more data were collected to provide better estimates of the group parameters, quantities could be calculated very easily which would have a straightforward interpretation and could be readily understood by medical personnel and which appear to discriminate between the different degrees of diabetes. In particular the posterior expectations of the excess glucose and excess C-peptide, which are, in a sense, updated version of the index of [3], appear to be potentially useful.

ACKNOWLEDGEMENT

We wish to express our thanks to Dr. L.S.P. Wickramasinghe and his co-authors for permission to use the data.

REFERENCES

[1] Wickramasinghe, L.S.P., Chazan, B.I., Farrow, M., Bansal, S.K. and Basu, S.K., "C-peptide Response to Oral Glucose and its Clinical Value in the Elderly", In submission.

[2] Ackerman E., Rosevear, J.W. and McGuckin, W.F., (1964), "A Mathematical Model of the Glucose-Tolerance Test", Physics in Medicine and Biology, **9**, 203-213.

[3] Billewicz, W.Z., Anderson, J. and Lind, T., (1973), "New Index for Evaluation of Oral Glucose Tolerance Test Results", British Medical Journal, **1**, 573-577.

[4] De Groot, M.H., (1970), "Optimal Statistical Decisions", McGraw-Hill, New York.

[5] Laird, N.M. and Ware, J.H., (1982), "Random Effects Models for Longitudinal Data", Biometrics, **38**, 963-974.

[6] Crowder, M.J. and Tredger, J.A., (1981), "The Use of Exponentially Damped Polynomials for Biological Recovery Data", Applied Statistics, **30**, 147-152.

[7] Crowder, M.J., (1983), "A Growth Curve Analysis for E.D.P. Curves", Applied Statistics, **32**, 15-18.

[8] Dempster, A.P., Rubin, D.B. and Tsutakawa, R.K., (1981), "Estimation in Covariance Components Models", Journal of the American Statistical Association", **76**, 341-353.